Contents

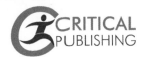
CRITICAL
PUBLISHING

PSYCHO
PHARMACOLOGY

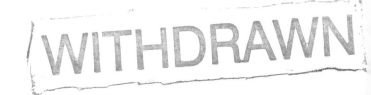
WITHDRAWN

A mental health professional's guide to commonly used medications

First published in 2018 by Critical Publishing Ltd

British Library Cataloguing in Publication Data
A CIP record for this book is available from the British Library

ISBN: 978-1-912096-04-6

This book is also available in the following e-book formats:

MOBI ISBN: 978-1-912096-03-9
EPUB ISBN: 978-1-912096-02-2
Adobe e-book ISBN: 978-1-912096-01-5

Cover design by Out of House Limited
Text design by Greensplash
Project Management by Out of House Publishing Solutions
Printed and bound in Great Britain by Bell & Bain, Glasgow

Critical Publishing
3 Connaught Road
St Albans
AL3 5RX

www.criticalpublishing.com

Meet the author

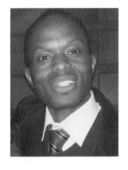 **Herbert Mwebe** is a lecturer in mental health in the School of Health and Education at Middlesex University. Within the department of mental health, Herbert delivers physical health training for both undergraduate and postgraduate programmes. He leads on continuing professional development courses focusing on developing mental health professionals' knowledge and skills in relation to improving physical health in serious mental illness and medication management in adult mental health settings.

Prior to entering academia, Herbert worked in both inpatient and community settings providing mental health care to people with serious mental illness; most recently in general practice, Herbert led on a mental health project in City and Hackney commissioned by NHS England to provide timely management of people presenting with mental illness in primary care.

Herbert also works with the Care Quality Commission (CQC) in the capacity of specialist clinical advisor, supporting CQC health and social care provider inspections.

Acknowledgements

In writing this book, I would like to acknowledge the following people.

Third-year mental health nursing students whose feedback in the earlier stages of this project provided valuable insight in the writing and planning of the book.

I am grateful to all those who kindly agreed to review the book, and especially Dr Geeta Patel for always providing me with personal and professional guidance.

Nobody has been more important to me in the pursuit of this project than the members of my family. I would like to thank my parents, whose love and guidance are with me in whatever I pursue. They are the ultimate role models. Most importantly, I wish to thank my loving and supportive wife, for her ongoing support and words of encouragement. Thank you for giving time to review and edit the book draft.

Finally, I would like to thank God, for without His presence in my life I would not be what I am today.

Herbert Mwebe

Foreword

I met Herbert in 2014, and at that time he was leading an innovative GP-based mental health project in a busy urban setting in East London, at the front line of psychiatric care and forming a vital bridge between primary and secondary mental health services.

Herbert brought his secondary care experience into the heart of primary care. He was located in the GP practices, seeing patients, advising the primary care team, bringing mental health expertise to where it was needed most. I was also working in that gap between primary and secondary care as a primary care liaison psychiatrist, and although I was secondary care mental health trust employed and Herbert was primary care employed, we had a similar ethos and worked together to care for patients.

I have been a consultant psychiatrist in East London since 2009 and took up the role of lead consultant for primary care liaison in 2015. Primary mental health care is vitally important, not just for common mental disorders and first-episode presentations to primary care professionals, but increasingly for long-term management of people with chronic but stable severe and enduring mental health problems discharged from secondary care services.

Herbert's skill in the assessment and management of mental health issues was readily apparent, and his wisdom in knowing when and how to intervene was invaluable. He was able to contain complex situations at the GP surgery, without referring and waiting for secondary care appointments. For patients, his input in the less stigmatising and more familiar environment of their family GP's surgery was hugely welcome. For GPs, having Herbert's knowledge and advice so readily available in the surgery was 'just what the doctor ordered'. He helped many patients through crises, not just with medication but providing holistic care and using psychosocial interventions with patients at the centre of their care. His real forte was in the management of physical health conditions in people with long-term mental health conditions. He reviewed the care of many patients on long-term depot antipsychotics who had been discharged back to primary care, making dose changes and ensuring physical health monitoring was prioritised. His expertise in balancing medication to optimise efficacy for mental health symptoms while minimising unwanted physical and metabolic side effects gave confidence to GPs to make dose reductions and substitutions, without the need for re-referral back to secondary care.

I remember a particular patient in his late 50s who had been on depot medication for more than 20 years, without the need for secondary care input for at least ten years, whose dose had not changed since his discharge from the psychiatry clinic. He had been invited to come to the surgery for annual reviews but had tended to avoid coming. He needed some encouragement and more assertive outreach. Herbert managed to engage with him and over a series of supportive contacts managed to get his co-operation in having physical health screening tests. An ECG picked up a significant issue with QT prolongation and Herbert spent several sessions with the patient discussing options and helping him to make an informed choice about his treatment. With the patient's wishes established, and with liaison discussions between myself, Herbert and the GP, we arranged for his depot to be reduced and stopped and to have a much lower dose of a different oral antipsychotic. The patient, having been invited to make active choices about his treatment, was more motivated to take the lead in decisions about his own recovery and later took up the offer of gym membership through 'exercise on prescription'. His GP felt supported and empowered to make decisions about longstanding antipsychotic medication, changes that the GP would have previously been hesitant to initiate without secondary care management.

It is no surprise, given the significant training aspect of his role in primary care, that Herbert went on to further develop his teaching portfolio, becoming a lecturer in mental health in the School of Health and Education at Middlesex University, where he focuses on physical health training and medication management on the undergraduate and post-graduate programs.

This useful and practical textbook provides a concise and informative resource covering the psychotropic medications most commonly used in clinical practice. Background information about neurotransmitters and the pharmacological mechanism of action is presented clearly, balanced with practical and clinical applications. It explores how medication can be used to help people presenting with mental health symptoms and, in keeping with Herbert's practice as a clinician, it demonstrates how medication is just one tool in a range of possible interventions. He keeps the patient at the centre, with case discussions and real-life case examples as well as a focus on safety.

The book will be helpful for anyone working at the front line of mental health care, in primary or secondary care, including GPs, junior doctors and psychiatrists, practice and mental health nurses and professionals working in liaison services. Those undertaking educational health courses with a mental health focus will find this book useful. The summary at the end of each chapter would be particularly useful for students and non-medical prescribers, with learning outcomes and study activities laid out as a useful revision aid. This is a book designed for clinical use, with an emphasis on physical health and the impact of prescribing not just on mental health symptoms but on all systems, considering a holistic approach.

I see this book as an essential learning tool and practical reminder for anyone treating people with mental health symptoms. It is firmly established on my bookshelf already.

Dr Caroline Methuen
Consultant Psychiatrist
East London NHS Foundation Trust

What the reviewers say

I would recommend this book to all mental health nurse prescribers, nurses and students. The book layout is brilliant with a concise summary and questions at the end of each chapter, which makes the reader reflect on the content read in each chapter. Case discussion makes it more interesting and enhances your knowledge of each group of medication. The book, with the study activities, is very well written and a very useful resource for practitioners and learners.

Dr Geeta Patel
GP with specialist interest in psychiatry
Latimer Health Centre, City and Hackney CCG

The author has clearly put a lot of work in to writing this book and I like the ethos, how medication is looked at as a tool and how a reduction of symptoms may allow for other work to take place. I think it is written in a way to allow difficult concepts to be visualised in a memorable way. I was struck by the amount of information in a short read. The author identifies key points and creatively depicts application in a care setting. I imagine if I was a nurse I would find it a useful resource, but I also think it would be useful for other professionals.

David Rogalski
Lead Pharmacist, Practice Based Mental Health Team
Camden and Islington NHS Foundation Trust

I recommend this informative, accessible and easy-to-read book to mental health professionals. It is a clear, concise summary of the use of psychotropic drugs that are commonly used in mental health settings. It is useful for people new to mental health and a good summary for people who are experienced in the field. It is clearly laid out and well researched. It clearly explains concepts such as the pathogenesis of different mental illnesses, neurotransmitters and the biochemistry and pharmacology of different medication. Herbert Mwebe has a great deal of experience in the front line of mental health in various settings including acute psychiatric wards. His years of experience are demonstrated in this book. It is clearly laid out with relevant case examples that are commonly experienced. Under each chapter a drug group is discussed with a summary of learning outcomes set out for the reader at the beginning. Common conditions are discussed for which the specific drug group is indicated, the mechanism of action as well as adverse effects and/or side effects associated with the drugs. I will recommend this book to my colleagues.

Dr Rachel Gibbons
Consultant Psychiatrist in Psychiatry and Psychotherapy
Barnet Enfield and Haringey NHS Mental Health Trust
Psychoanalyst - Institute of Psychoanalysis

A very well written and well laid out piece. An easy read even for beginners.

Anu Patel
Community Pharmacist
Newcare Pharmacy, North West London

This comprehensive resource covers all the commonly used psychotropic drugs in detail, so that readers are fully informed; yet explains things in a clear, memorable and easy-to-understand way. I particularly like the case studies and end of chapter summaries and review questions, which will be very useful for students as a revision aid, but they also provide a succinct refresher for any practising health professional involved in the care of people with mental health disorders. This is a useful learning resource for all students or qualified health professionals (registered nurses, social workers, psychologists, pharmacists and doctors).

Dr Danielle Roberts
GP Specialist Trainee
Health Education England London Deanery

The primary purpose of this book is to inform the reader about the clinical use of psychiatric drugs. It assumes a user-friendly style, with consideration given to learning, revision and testing at the end of each chapter.

The key aspects of psychotropic drugs, their mechanisms of action and safe use are covered, with signposting to drug properties, such as additional safety netting requirements. Clinical applications are supported via useful case studies.

One of the strengths of this book is the patient-centred focus. This has the additional advantage of encouraging an holistic social and medical approach, which is essential to treat and promote mental health. By providing insight into the impact of these drugs upon the individual and into the range of systems to be considered when assessing and managing a patient on psychotropic medications, the reader is able to envisage the whole model of care.

This text should be useful for people at the beginning of their professional journey, as well as for clinicians who require additional knowledge about a psychotropic drug class, or for people undertaking a prescribing course.

Dr Sharon Rees
Associate Professor in Therapeutics and Prescribing
London Southbank University

Introduction

The main aim of this book is to provide mental health professionals with practical advice and knowledge of psychotropic drugs commonly used in clinical settings. The medications covered in this book are those recommended for adults presenting with a mental health disorder. The setting for use of this resource varies from community mental health teams, inpatient units, forensic services, primary care and/or residential care settings. This book can be used by a novice learner to the more advanced practitioner working independently in adult care settings such as inpatient wards, crisis and home treatment teams, liaison teams, community mental health recovery teams and as a reference for independent prescribers. The information contained in this book is based on literature review and clinical experience. The link between theory and practice is explicitly demonstrated in the different sections of the book. I do not claim that this information is necessarily more accurate compared to other literature or professional agencies. I hope, however, that this resource will be consulted alongside other similar resources to develop your understanding of commonly used medications in mental health settings and the monitoring of adverse effects caused by pharmacological agents. While I have tried to ensure that all indicated drug doses are accurate, health professionals should always consult statutory guidance and local and/or national prescribing formularies (eg the British National Formulary [BNF] or equivalent) before making any prescribing or medication administrative decisions. Every clinical presentation should always be treated and assessed on an individual basis and a thorough comprehensive mental, physical, psychological and social health assessment of needs must inform any clinical decisions. Furthermore, as this is an educational resource, some of the discussions may not meet UK licensing uses of some medications. Where necessary, I have indicated those medications that are only available on the US market and not in the UK.

This book benefits pre-registration mental health nursing students to meet the Nursing and Midwifery Council (NMC) competencies regarding medication management and monitoring of adverse effects of medications. The NMC announced this year that the current medicine management standards will be permanently withdrawn, but the regulator is working with the key stakeholders including the Royal Pharmaceutical Society (RPS) to help develop an ideal model or future guidance on medicines management and administration. Preparation in developing medicine management knowledge and skills so that patients receive better and safer care, and supporting health professionals and patients to make best use of medicines, is a required competence and is a necessity for acceptance and entry onto the NMC register as a mental health nurse. This resource will help the registered mental health nurse in meeting the NMC knowledge competence and required standards on safe medication management and administration. Although this book will mostly benefit those students on the mental health nursing pathway, students on other health pathways in nursing will also find it beneficial in developing awareness and knowledge around medications commonly used in adult mental health settings. Registered nurses will find this book a useful resource for reference when undertaking continuing professional development courses (CPD), such as advanced nurse practitioner courses, non-medical prescribing modular courses and refresher study days on medication management in mental health settings. All this is relevant and can be used as evidence for professional development and for the revalidation process (NMC, 2015).

The author accepts no liability for any injury, loss or damage caused.

THE STRUCTURE OF THIS BOOK

Each chapter discusses a specific medication group, with a summary of learning outcomes set out at the beginning. The chapter then examines common conditions for which the specific medication group is indicated, the mechanism of action, and adverse effects and/or side effects associated with the drugs including common management approaches to lessen the burden of harm linked to unwanted effects caused by psychotropic medications. Common medication routes of administration are described and, where relevant, precautions to consider in clinical practice are discussed in relation to the use of psychotropic medications. A summary of the main key points is provided as a review of the chapter content covered to encourage reflection.

LEARNING FEATURES

Feedback provided by third year mental health nursing students on learning and teaching around psychopharmacological interventions included insights into the most effective layout for the book and useful learning features. These have been included.

Learning outcomes are provided at the beginning of each chapter to highlight what the reader can expect to have accomplished after working through the content of the chapter including the learning activities within it.

Case studies are a good way to help the reader to link theoretical knowledge around psychopharmacological interventions to day-to-day practice. Such practice may be undertaken in the assessment and clinical care management of people with mental illness exposed to psychotropic medications. The case studies in this book promote reflection on practice and highlight the central role mental health professionals play in the risk management and monitoring of patients in mental health settings.

A chapter summary with clear key points is provided as a brief snapshot of the chapter content to draw the reader's attention to key points in the chapter.

End of **chapter review questions** are provided to test the reader's understanding and to encourage reflective practice. Answers to these are given in the Appendix. The study questions provided are useful for the learner revising for exams or in planning study group discussions with other learners. Equally, they can be used by mental health professionals to refresh clinical knowledge and skills in relation to the safe use of psychopharmacological interventions in practice aimed at meeting required obligatory safe practices and/or guidelines in their respective clinical environments.

To help you navigate each chapter, below are some of the main headings used in each chapter (except for Chapter 1):

- Chapter aims
- Introduction
- Mechanism of action
- Dosage and administration
- Adverse effects and management
- Chapter summary
- Case study
- Review questions

1 Mental illness

CHAPTER AIMS

This chapter covers:

- the brief history of psychiatric drugs and alternative interventions used in mental health settings;
- the aetiology of mental illness;
- neurodevelopment and biochemical theories implicated in the aetiology of mental illness;
- the most common neurotransmitters, their role and function;
- the role of mental health nurses, prescribers and others in medication management;
- clinical decision-making in mental health nursing.

1.1 INTRODUCTION

Psychiatric medicine as well as contemporary mental health nursing heavily relies on psychotropic drugs. The phrase 'psychotropic drugs' is a technical term for psychiatric medicines that alter chemical levels in the brain which impact on mood and behaviour. Medications can play a role in treating many mental illnesses and conditions. Psychiatric drugs have been available for more than six decades; also referred to as neuroleptic drugs, they are used to treat and manage symptoms of organic psychoses and mania. Psychiatric drugs just like any other medication have side effects, ranging from minor to more complex and serious adverse effects for the patient. There is now a well-established body of evidence relating to the effects and past as well as current research has focused on the health implications of consuming these pharmaceutical agents. Psychiatric drug use in clinical settings has indeed revolutionised the understanding around theory and practice of mental health nursing. The mental health nurse's role in the monitoring of side effects of psychiatric drugs is therefore a vital step of the patient's care plan. Firstly, the nurse must be able to identify and evaluate side effects of the medication because the side effects may mirror the symptoms of mental conditions; this could present challenges in developing a clearly focused care plan for the patient in relation to their specific needs identified and aligning these with the necessary and most effective interventions.

Medicines are usually more effective when combined with alternative interventions for people with mental illness; these might include but are not limited to cognitive behavioural therapy (CBT), counselling, interpersonal therapy, family therapy, psychoeducation, healthy eating, sleep hygiene, empathetic listening, problem solving, exercise and budgeting. In some cases, medication can reduce symptoms so that other methods of interventions in care planning can become more effective. It is important to explore the usefulness of all interventions (pharmacological and psychosocial treatment strategies) when considering care planning and to not focus on a single intervention. For instance, a commonly used antidepressant called sertraline may lessen some significant symptoms of major depression and CBT may help the patient to change negative attitudes and patterns of thinking. Predicting patient response to medication is not always straightforward as some medications could work better for one person than for another (National Institute for Health and Care Excellence [NICE], 2018b). Prescribers (doctors, nurses and/or pharmacists) should review clinical literature and clinical records to see if there is evidence for recommending one type of medicine over another. For example, mirtazapine, a common antidepressant, may be preferred over citalopram when there is problematic chronic insomnia; this is because it has been shown to enhance sedation and sleep even at lower doses compared to citalopram. Various factors should be considered by prescribers when planning pharmacological interventions, ie side effects, family history, existing physical health conditions, contra-indications, a patient's concordance to medication, lifestyle behaviours, allergies and consideration for other drugs (prescribed or recreational) the patient may be taking. The mental health nurse, by working alongside medical and non-medical prescribers, must ensure that patients receiving psychopharmacological interventions are closely monitored in relation to safe medication usage and management.

It is not unusual for the patient to try more than one drug at the initiation of treatment to establish the most appropriate drug; factors such as the patient's symptom profile, side effects and any past or previous response to other drugs should form part of the initial assessment. Patient involvement and active participation in the process of decision-making is vital to create a collaborative working partnership between the healthcare professional and the patient. The success of this shared care partnership is vital for the development of effective care plans. Family members and other carers should also be included in these discussions if the patient gives their consent.

Some drugs used in mental health settings work quickly. For example, lorazepam, which is commonly used for short-term treatment and management of anxiety, produces a calming effect and improvement in patients can be evident within hours. Other drugs may have a slow onset of action, requiring some patients to take the medication for several weeks before any improvement is seen. Medication therapy may be a short-term treatment strategy in which medications may be taken for a few weeks to months. In other cases, medication therapy may be a long-term or even life-long treatment strategy. Patients may be afraid that consuming medication may change their personality and lives; however, most patients find that taking the medication allows them to take charge of their situation and enables them to become more independent and actively participate in care planning to further improve their quality of life.

1.2 AETIOLOGY OF MENTAL ILLNESS

Mental illness can arise from many different sources. To date, there is no single confirmed or reliable accepted cause established. A common belief is that mental illness arises when genetic vulnerabilities and environmental factors interact, with the latter often acting as a catalyst to expose genetic vulnerabilities. This model has been theorised explicitly by the diathesis-stress model (Sullivan, 2009) and similarly the stress-vulnerability model proposed by Zubin and Spring (1977). To put it simply, when stress factors (eg bereavement, poverty, loss of employment, complex interpersonal dynamics) and vulnerability (ie genetic, chronic physical illness, stressful life events) interact beyond a threshold, mental illness emerges. People with traumatic brain injuries are at greater risk of developing mental health related conditions, and environmental factors surrounding pregnancy and birth complications have also been implicated. Though, it is conceivable that the pregnancy and birth complications may reflect rather than cause mental illness. There is also wider acknowledgement of a strong relationship between complex mental illness in adults and abuse (physical, emotional, sexual) and psychological trauma in early years. As such, psychosocial and interpersonal theories have also become a focus of recovery-orientated strategies to understand how factors such as environmental, social, economic and upbringing may affect the course of mental illness.

Research has shown that genes play an important role in the development of mental illness but there has been little progress linking specific genes to specific mental health conditions. It has traditionally been assumed that changes in DNA structure is exclusively accountable for the development of schizophrenia. However, twin studies show that it is also conceivable that an epigenetic mechanism may contribute to the development of schizophrenia. Genetic contribution to the course of mental illness is significant and has been demonstrated by twin, family and adoption studies (Duncan et al, 2004; Gejman et al, 2010). In relation to schizophrenia and twin studies, a concordance rate of around 45–50 per cent has been reported for monozygotic twins, compared to only a 10–15 per cent concordance rate for fraternal twins. This commonly cited evidence in a wider body of literature is largely considered the most significant piece of evidence supporting the biological theory of schizophrenia and seen as modest proof underpinning this theory relating to the course of schizophrenia (Joseph, 2003; Rapp et al, 2003). However, the lack of 100 per cent concordance rates in monozygotic twins is also evidence that aetiology is not entirely genetic.

While the cause of depression has not been fully established, several theories have been reported in the pathophysiology of depression. Genetic contribution has been established with twin studies indicating that certain presentations of depressive disorder appear to be genetic. There is a reported increase in risk of bipolar disorder in the relatives of patients with bipolar disorder. Relatives of both bipolar and unipolar patients are also at increased risk of unipolar depression (Cuellar et al, 2005). Previous history of a mental illness (depression, schizophrenia, bipolar disorder) may increase the risk of further episodes. Major depressive disorder is also two to three times more common in women; similarly, unipolar depression in women is double that seen in males (Blows, 2011).

Psychoanalytic theories have also been proposed to explain the cause of mental illness. To this end, the theories offer rationality in relation to unresolved internal and interpersonal relational conflicts. Similarly, the attachment theory, which is often applied to understanding psychopathology, is informed by evolutionary psychology approaches that focus on the role early object relations play, ie early care giver–child relationships, and uncovering any tensions (anger, frustration, resentment) and the need to find satisfying positive object relations in adult life. Psychoanalytic theorists incorporate and assimilate the biopsychosocial model in their approach. The biopsychosocial model is now commonly used in the western world but while it emphasises the biological, social and psychological entities with regards to understanding aetiology of disease and illness, psychiatric care in the west continues to be mostly dominated by the medical model (disease model). Distinctions are commonly made between the disease model (focusing on symptoms, absence of symptoms) and social model (recovery model) of mental illness, which aims to homogenise the biopsychosocial understanding of psychopathology by focusing on social derivatives and constructions.

Biochemical theories implicate abnormalities in neurotransmitter circuit systems of dopamine, glutamate, serotonin, gamma-aminobutyric acid (GABA), adrenaline/noradrenalin and acetylcholine in the causes of mental illness. The next sub-sections look at this in more detail.

1.3 NEURODEVELOPMENTAL THEORIES

Neurodevelopmental theories are supported by abnormalities in the physiology of the brain, its structures and functions in the post-mortem of patients with schizophrenia. When reporting abnormalities, neuro-scientists have discovered both structural and functional changes, ie enlarged lateral and third cerebral ventricles (cavities in the brain filled with cerebrospinal fluid [CSF]) and decrease in whole brain volume are consistent findings. Patients with schizophrenia, including people who have never been treated, have a reduced volume of grey matter in the brain, especially in the temporal and frontal lobes, hippocampus, amygdala and parahippocampal gyrus. Neuroscientists have found grey matter loss of up to 25 per cent in some regions of the brain. The loss, which had started in the parietal or outer regions of the brain, had spread to the rest of the brain over a five-year period. The patients with most brain tissue loss also had the worst symptoms; including hallucinations, delusions, bizarre and psychotic thoughts, hearing voices and depression (Hata et al, 2003; Brent et al, 2013). Suggested associations between reduced frontal lobe activity and negative (affective) symptoms commonly exhibited by patients have been reported as well as associations linking positive symptoms (delusions, auditory hallucinations) and increases in regional cerebral blood flow in brain language areas (Duncan et al, 2004; Castelnovo et al, 2015).

Neurons and neurotransmitters

The central nervous system (CNS) controls most functions of the body and mind. It consists of two parts: the brain and the spinal cord. The brain is central to thoughts, emotions, behaviours, understanding and interpreting our external environment, muscle and motor control. Neurons and neurotransmitters play a significant role in moderating all these body processes and thus contribute to our daily well-being. There are between 30–100 neurotransmitter molecule types, with ten of these doing 99 per cent of the work. Neuroscientific research has mainly focused on the following main categories of neurotransmitters: glutamate, GABA, dopamine, serotonin, noradrenaline, acetylcholine, and histamine (National Institute of Mental Health, 2016; Whishaw et al, 2016). Abnormalities in these biochemical neurotransmitter circuit systems of the brain has been the focus of neuroscience research.

Neurons (or nerve cells) are the functional units of the CNS; neurotransmitters are chemical messengers between one neuron to another. The neurotransmitters carry impulses (messages) between neurons at specific junctions called synapses. All nerve impulses or chemical reactions originate within the neuron. Impulses resulting from neurotransmitter transmission travel along the axon of the nerve to initiate one of many actions inside or outside the brain, for example:

- triggering another nerve impulse;
- a muscle contraction;
- a glandular secretion.

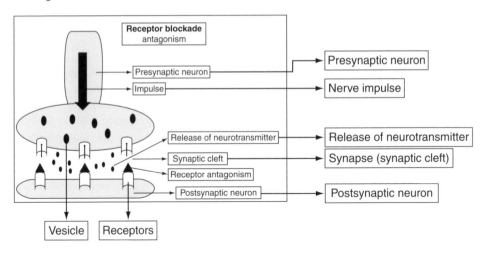

Figure 1.1 Neurons and neurotransmitter mechanism

In the above illustration (Figure 1.1), the onset of a nerve impulse excites the release of neurotransmitters from vesicles. The released neurotransmitter travels across the presynaptic nerve cell membrane to the synapse. The neurotransmitters pass across the synaptic cleft or synapse, bind to special molecules (proteins) called receptors and open channels located on the postsynaptic neuron of the target organ/muscle/nerve cell. The charged particles subsequently enter and trigger a second impulse. This process happens with quick precision and is repeated as the signal or impulse is passed at split-second speed from neuron to neuron (Südhof, 2004). The mechanism by which the neuron releases neurotransmitters has been the focus of considerable research. Scientists found that neurotransmitters are stored in small, bubble-like

Table 1.1 A summary of neurotransmitter types and effects in the body

Neurotransmitter	Key role	Effects of increased	Effects of reduced
Serotonin (excitatory & inhibitory)	Inhibits behaviour and activity, enhances sleep time, temperature regulation, pain perception and mood states	Induces sedation, but if significantly raised can result in mania and hallucinations	Depression, sleep disturbances, irritability and hostile behaviour
Dopamine (excitatory)	Decision-making, thinking, fine muscle movements, integration of emotions and thought processes	Loose associations, disorganised thoughts, stereotypical behaviours, tics and psychosis	Parkinson's disease and movement disorders, depression, fatigue, mood swings
GABA (inhibitory)	Balances and regulates excitatory neurons, regulates and restricts neuroelectric activity and involved in allergies	Excessive drowsiness may induce narcolepsy	Difficulty thinking or concentrating, tremors, stress, loss of motor control, personality changes, anxiety
Noradrenaline (excitatory and inhibitory)	Alertness, capacity to focus, attention, capacity to be orientated, fight or flight (sympathetic response)	Loss of appetite, hypervigilance, anxiety, paranoia	Low energy, dull feeling, depression, low blood pressure, lethargy, inattention
Adrenaline (excitatory)	Adrenal medulla releases adrenaline. Adrenaline causes many physiological changes to prepare the body for fight or flight (eg increased heart rate, pupil dilation, etc)	Paranoia, mania, weight loss or gain, muscle weakness, depression, anxiety, fatigue, sleep disturbances, excess facial and body hair and/or irregular periods in women	Low energy, dull feeling, depression, fatigue, loss of appetite

(continued)

Table 1.1 (*Cont.*)

Neurotransmitter	Key role	Effects of increased	Effects of reduced
Acetylcholine (excitatory)	Stimulates muscles, helps in memory function, activates pain responses and regulates endocrine secretions	Self-consciousness, over inhibition, depression, psycho-somatic complaints and anxiety	Anticholinergic effects (eg dry mouth, blurred vision), lack of inhibition, poor memory, euphoria, parkinsonism, antisocial behaviour, speech problems, manic behaviour
Glutamate (major excitatory neurotransmitter; N-methyl-D-aspartate [NMDA] receptors)	Involved in typical metabolic functions like energy production and ammonia purification in addition to protein synthesis. Neural communication, memory formation, learning, thinking and regulation	Increased levels of glutamate over-stimulation leads to further neural death/degeneration, which results in poor memory function/learning Alzheimer's disease	Glutamatergic abnormalities are implicated in schizophrenia due to hypofunction of glutamatergic systems

cubicles called vesicles. Each vesicle will usually hold a single type of neurotransmitter, such as dopamine, which is associated with memory and other cognitive skills, or serotonin, which helps regulate mood, appetite and aids in digestion. The vesicles travel like foot soldiers towards the end of the discharging neuron where they dock, waiting to be released through the synapse to eventually bind to the receptors of the receiving neuron. After the neurotransmitter binds with the receptor (a site on the postsynaptic nerve cell), the neurotransmitter can either produce two effects: (1) exciting or stimulating the receiving neuron or organ, or (2) inhibition (dampening or blocking action) on the postsynaptic neuron activity. The neurotransmitter breaks away from the receptor and is either recycled back (re-uptake) into the releasing neuron by a neurotransmitter responder or deactivated by enzymes in the synaptic space (Südhof and Rothman, 2009). Following neurotransmitter release, the neuron recycles the empty vesicles, refilling and reusing them several more times before they are replaced. Changes in functioning of any part of this process – if a neuron fails to do its job properly or if the vesicles release their neurotransmitters at the wrong speed – can result in the development of serious problems. Scientists have discovered that in the brains of people with depression, serotonin, which is responsible for regulating mood and enabling sleep, is low and not transmitted effectively between brain nerves. It is proposed that alteration in the level of function within these neurotransmitters may offer understanding of the pathogenesis of some psychiatric disorders, such as schizophrenia, depression, anxiety states, attention deficit hyperactivity disorder (ADHD), mood disorders and other neurodegenerative conditions such as dementia and parkinsonism.

Each neurotransmitter has one or two important roles at the receptor sites; the neurotransmitter either has an excitatory or inhibitory effect or both. Neurotransmitter role and function may include regulating bodily functions such as thinking, feelings, motor and sensory activity, thermoregulation, behavioural control, digestion etc.

1.4 CLINICAL DECISION-MAKING IN PRACTICE AND MEDICINE MANAGEMENT

Mental health professionals play a critical role in meeting patients' need and promoting care that is of high quality and safe. For example, the Nursing Midwifery Council (NMC) professional code of conduct stipulates that registered nurses are accountable for providing, leading and co-ordinating nursing care tailored to a person's needs and to be compassionate (NMC, 2015). To achieve this, nurses must work collaboratively and involve patients and partner with various healthcare professionals to meet the health care needs and informed by the most current evidence (Mwebe, 2017; NMC, 2017). The way in which healthcare is provided has undergone various changes since the inception of the National Health Service (NHS) in the late 1940s. Healthcare professionals work in continued cultures of change against a backdrop of challenging environments, growing diversity and rapidly ever-changing complexity of patient needs. The Australian Public Service commission report (2007) used the term 'wicked' in relation to complex societal and individual determinants of health which are often difficult to define and are caused by factors of varying degrees. For example, unhealthy lifestyle behaviours such as smoking, drug and alcohol abuse, unhealthy eating and sedentary lifestyles are significantly more prevalent in people with mental illness than in people without mental illness (Dunstan, 2010; Szatkowsk et al, 2015 BIB). In particular, people with serious mental illness smoke significantly more, have increased levels of nicotine dependency and are therefore at even greater risk of smoking-related harm (Office for National Statistics, 2016; Mental Health Foundation, 2016). Consequently, it is unsurprising that people with serious mental illness die on average 10–20 years earlier than people without mental illness (Action on Smoking and Health, 2018). Among other factors, this disparity is often due to low emphasis on strategies to screen for physical health problems in people with mental illness and inadequate targeted practices such as monitoring for adverse effects of psychotropic drugs and screening for unhealthy lifestyle behaviours (Mwebe, 2017). The rates of metabolic syndrome (a risk factor for developing cardiovascular disease [CVD], diabetes, stroke) are reported to be as high as 60 per cent in people with serious mental illness (Crump et al, 2013).

It is therefore important that mental health professionals providing care for people accessing mental health services are equipped with the right knowledge and skills and are confident to participate in the necessary decision-making processes in practice to respond to complex and diverse needs of patients. The NMC (2015) expects mental health trainee nurses and registered mental health nurses to act with professionalism, communicate and exhibit relationship building skills when undertaking nursing procedures and clinical decisions needed to screen and respond to patients at risk. Mutsatsa (2015) argues that the nurse must ensure that any clinical decision made considers the patient at the centre of their care with emphasis on a shared decision-making process between the nurse and the patient to promote shared learning and trust. The ability to reflect and think critically, apply skills and knowledge and deliver specialist nursing care interventions in areas such as medicine management and physical health care therefore lies at the forefront of pre-registration nursing education programmes and equally is a bedrock for all nursing practice. However, mental health nurses' knowledge and skills regarding pharmacological interventions and link to practice has been questioned in research studies (Offredy et al, 2008) and by nurses themselves (Bradley et al, 2006). It is unsurprising that Mwebe (2017) found varying levels of practice and knowledge among inpatient mental health nurses in relation to physical health care needs of people with mental illness. Mental health nursing education in the UK is now more inclusive in that physical health training at both undergraduate and postgraduate levels is becoming part of the curriculum so that registered nurses and student nurses are trained and equipped with the necessary knowledge and skills to be ready and prepared to tackle physical health and other concerns in serious mental illness. All this is vital to empower mental health nurses to confidently make appropriate clinical decisions in practice. For example, mental health nurse prescribers may consider reflecting on the following questions when consulting and preparing a prescription for their patient.

- What is the therapeutic effect of the medication? Is it necessary and/or appropriate?
- What is the past and current medical history?
- What are the alternatives?
- What is the patient's view of the clinical benefits of the drug?
- What is the patient's experience?
- What are the patient's expectations from treatment?
- Is there a conflict and do you feel under pressure to prescribe?
- Is there problematic recreational drug use?
- What physical health co-morbidities must I consider?
- What level of engagement is needed to ensure the patient is an active partner in their care planning?

The new pre-registration education and practice standards published by the NMC (2017) reflect the future/current needs of the public for expert nursing care; the revamped educational framework for training nurses in the UK have been developed to reflect these needs. The educational standards propose the future nurse should generally be ready and prepared to meet patient and service needs and that at the point of qualifying, nurses should be ready to work in a range of sectors and specialties to provide a high quality of care. Among the pre-registration education changes proposed in relation to preparatory nursing training is to develop and increase the knowledge and skills of nurses around effective non-medical prescribing and exit higher education training with a wide range of clinical skills (Royal Pharmaceutical Society, 2016). For mental health trainee nurses this requires a sound knowledge of the pathology of mental illness, assessment and risk management and pharmacotherapeutics. In practice, decisions to treat symptoms related to mental illness are not taken lightly and often involve a multidisciplinary team approach to plan for various patient needs including social, environmental, biological and psychological. The future mental health nurse or mental health prescriber must not only appreciate the impact of these factors on a person's health but exercise awareness of different interventions and safely apply these to individual cases, adopting a person-centred approach. In particular, decision-making in practice around psychopharmacological interventions requires a sound understanding of pharmacodynamics and kinetics of how psychotropic drugs work in the body and the obligatory monitoring measures to ensure drugs are used safely in line with the current evidence base, clinical guidelines and statutory frameworks to minimise risk of harm to patients. The clinical decisions made by mental health professionals (mental health nurses, social workers, psychologists, psychiatrists) have significant implications on the patient. It is therefore a professional obligation for clinicians to engage, evaluate and incorporate evidence in their day-to-day clinical decision-making and professional judgement.

The Medicines and Healthcare Products Regulatory Agency (MHRA, 2008) defines medicine management as '*the clinical, cost-effective and safe use of medicines to ensure patients get the maximum benefit from the medicines they need, while at the same time minimising potential harm*'. Similarly, the standards for medicine management clearly state that all registered nurses must possess the necessary knowledge and leadership skills to inform the prescriber without delay where adverse effects and contra-indications to prescribed medicines are found or when patients develop a reaction to the medicine (NMC, 2015b). Currently the NMC is collaboratively working with the Royal Pharmaceutical Society as they review and update their guidance entitled 'Professional Guidance on Safe and Secure Handling of Medicines in all Care Settings'. It is expected that this could benefit and provide an ideal model for future guidance on medicines management and administration (NMC, 2018). Mental health professionals are responsible for opportunistic screening and continued assessment of patients under their care. As antipsychotic drugs can cause significant physiological changes leading to poor physical health outcomes in patients, mental health nurses have continued responsibility for recognising and acting upon any changes in the patient's physiological parameters. The management and assessment of risk to promote the safe use of medicines should involve a clear and responsive model of inter and intraprofessional working partnerships. The NMC Essential Skills Clusters developed about nurses' fitness to practice at the point of registration emphasise mandatory requirements that pre-registration nurses must demonstrate competency in the medicine administration and calculation domain. Currently, facilitating of student nurse learning and assessment in practice is undertaken by suitably registered mental health nurses to prepare student nurses with the right attitude, skills and knowledge to be able to meet NMC pre-registration requirements. While this role under the new NMC practice learning standards is expected to be undertaken by registered nurses and other suitably qualified health professionals, for mental health nursing students in practice, a collaborative effort from different healthcare professionals contributing to the learning and assessment of students is most welcome. Facilitating learning could involve, among other roles, developing the trainee nurse's knowledge and confidence to recognise the most commonly used psychiatric drugs, side effects and recommended monitoring. The example below shows a typical learning scenario in relation to medication administration linking theoretical learning to practice.

Case study 1 – Medication administration

Background

Rose is a second-year mental health nursing student on her third week into a clinical placement on an inpatient mental health unit. Rose has started the morning shift and has been asked to observe a consultation between the junior doctor on the ward and Tom who was admitted to the unit the previous night. Tom has a diagnosis of paranoid schizophrenia. The consultation is in relation to a medication review as it had been alleged by the patient's community mental health team that Tom had stopped taking the medication prescribed to him. On this occasion, Tom is agreeable to resume taking his medication; the doctor starts the patient on olanzapine which is an atypical antipsychotic drug commonly used in mental health settings. The doctor also prescribes other drugs (haloperidol and lorazepam) that can be used as and when required on the reverse side of Tom's medication chart. Later that day, Tom becomes aroused and agitated in presentation; the team try non-pharmacological de-escalation techniques to manage Tom's presentation but to little effect. The team decide to offer Tom a dose of haloperidol 5 mg and 2 mg of lorazepam to take orally. Tom agrees and takes the medication. A few hours later, Tom reports to Rose that he is experiencing dizziness, light-headedness, drowsiness, headache and muscle stiffness.

Clinical decision-making process (linking theory to practice)

Rose immediately recalls theory from a university lecture that antipsychotic medications can induce unwanted physiological effects when administered to patients. Rose offers one-to-one support to Tom and reassures him that the effects reported are likely to be caused by haloperidol, which had been administered to Tom earlier. Given her level of training and experience, Rose informs the nurse in charge about the situation and her own interpretations. The nurse in charge confirms and agrees with Rose and she explains to Tom that the side effects are related to haloperidol, which is known for inducing extrapyramidal side effects, including muscle spasm/stiffness, shaking/tremor, restlessness, mask-like facial expression and drooling. The nurse in charge offers another medication called procyclidine, which is used in clinical settings to mitigate against extrapyramidal side effects induced by mostly older antipsychotic drugs, eg haloperidol, chlorpromazine.

The nurse in charge informs Tom that dizziness and light-headedness can increase the risk of falling, so Tom is advised by both the nurse and Rose to get up slowly when rising from a sitting or lying position. Rose offers to carry out a set of vital signs checks to assess any changes in blood pressure, pulse and respiratory parameters. Due to the risk of falls, the nurse in charge requests a support assistant to stay with Tom for the remainder of the shift to monitor for any further changes in presentation to ensure Tom's safety while he remains under the care of the ward. The junior doctor is informed about Tom's situation and offers to assess the patient at the next available opportunity but advises the nursing team to not administer haloperidol any further. In Chapter 2, extrapyramidal side effects and other effects associated with the use of antipsychotic medications are covered in detail.

The events in this scenario also demonstrate the opportunity and the need for a multidisciplinary team (MDT) working approach. A MDT is a partnership of specialised and non-specialised social and healthcare professionals who have distinctly different skills, knowledge and expertise, yet work together towards the common goal of providing the best patient care across variable services. The MDT is inextricably connected to the shared objective of providing effective care interventions (screening, monitoring, follow up) and overall care management to promote patients' health and well-being. Pharmacists among others (social workers, psychologists, occupational therapists, activity workers, independent mental health advocates) form part of the wider MDT in both inpatient and community mental health teams. In this scenario, the junior doctor, the registered nurse and the student nurse may consider involving a pharmacist who may provide further advice to address any medication management issues arising from Tom's care.

Generally, to aid clinical decision-making in practice regarding medication management, healthcare professionals have access to and may refer to the following resources at their disposal:

- *The Maudsley Prescribing Guidelines in Psychiatry.*
- *British National Formulary (BNF).*
- *Local NHS Trust Prescribing Formulary.*
- *National Institute for Health and Care Excellence Clinical Guidelines.*
- *The Nursing and Midwifery Council Standards for Medicines Management.*
- *The Mental Health Act 1983 as amended by the 2007 Act.*
- *United Kingdom Teratology Information Service.*
- *Medicines and Healthcare Products Regulatory Agency (Antipsychotics e-learning module).*
- *The electronic Medicines Compendium (eMC) contains up-to-date, easily accessible information about medicines licensed for use in the UK.*
- *The NHS Specialist Pharmacy Service (SPS) supports medicines optimisation across the NHS.*
- *MIND (mental health charity).*
- *HeadMeds, gives young people in the UK general information about medication.*
- *Choice and Medication and NHS 24 provide advice on mental health conditions and medications.*
- *Royal Pharmaceutical Society's Competency Framework for all Prescribers (RPS, 2016).*
- *Medicine Act 1968.*
- *Local medicine management policy.*
- *Local physical health policy.*
- *Rapid tranquilisation policy.*

CHAPTER SUMMARY

Key points

- Psychiatric drugs are the mainstay for the treatment and management of moderate to severe mental illness, but the use of psychiatric drugs should not define the role of mental health professionals.
- Treatment and management of mental illness involves a wide range of interventions; these include psychotropic drugs, CBT, counselling, interpersonal therapy, family therapy, psychoeducation, healthy eating, sleep hygiene, empathetic listening, problem solving, exercise, budgeting and others.
- The aetiology of mental illness is an interplay of genetic factors, neurodevelopmental and biochemical abnormalities and environmental factors including social and interpersonal interactions playing a role.
- Biochemical theories implicate abnormalities in the neurotransmitter systems of the brain, ie dopamine, serotonin, noradrenaline, glutamate, GABA, acetylcholine in the aetiology of mental illness.

- Mental health nurses and others must exercise vigilance in addressing various needs of the patient and be up-to-date in knowledge and skills to make appropriate clinical decisions when assessing and monitoring people with mental illness; most importantly, patients who are exposed to psychopharmacological interventions.

CHAPTER 1 REVIEW QUESTIONS

Now have a go at answering these questions. You might find it useful to refer to the content of the chapter to locate the correct information for each question.

1. What are antipsychotic medications?

2. What other name is usually used to refer to antipsychotic drugs?

3. What is the stress-vulnerability model and how does it contribute to the understanding behind the aetiology of mental illness?

4. What is a neuron? Give another name for a neuron.

5. Where do nerve impulses or chemical reactions originate from?

6. What is the space between two neurons called?

7. What do you call the cubicles where neurotransmitters are found?

8. What is the main difference between the presynaptic and postsynaptic neuron?

9. Give an example of a neurotransmitter.

10. Dopamine is found in the brain. True or false?

11. If someone has low serotonin levels in their brain, what are the likely health implications?

12. To understand how psychotropic medicines work, it is important to understand the theory behind neurotransmitter pathways and mechanisms in the brain. True or false?

13. What are the likely health effects of having low glutamate?

14. In Alzheimer's disease, low_____neurotransmitter is likely to lead to poor memory. Fill in the missing word.

15. What does CNS stand for?

16. What might be the effects of having too much glutamate?

17. What might be the effects of having too much dopamine?

18. Name one excitatory and one inhibitory neurotransmitter.

19. The genetic contribution of genes has been demonstrated by what type of studies?

20. What are the clinical uses of lorazepam?

21. There are approximately between_____neurotransmitter molecule types, with_____of them doing 99 per cent of the work. Fill in the missing words.

22. The loss of motor control and changes in personality may occur when there is a lack of what neurotransmitter?

23. Impulses resulting from neurotransmitter transmission travel in the nerve cell may initiate one of many actions inside or outside the brain. Give examples of the actions.

24. What might be the effects of excess serotonin?

25. Give two examples of neurodegenerative conditions.

26. What is the relationship between neurotransmitters and vesicles?

27. What factors should be considered by psychiatrists and mental health nurse prescribers when preparing a prescription of psychotropic drugs?

28. What does CBT stand for? Give a brief description.

29. What condition could result from having low dopamine?

30. In the case scenario about Tom, which medication is responsbile for him experiencing dizziness, light-headedness, drowsiness, headache and muscle stiffness?

2 Drugs used in psychoses

CHAPTER AIMS

This chapter covers:

- the symptomatology of schizophrenia;
- the glutamate and dopamine hypotheses of schizophrenia;
- the mechanism of action of antipsychotic drugs;
- different groups and types of antipsychotic drugs used in mental health settings;
- the adverse effects associated with antipsychotics;
- recommended monitoring and management of drug side effects;
- predisposing factors for the incidence of weight gain in the psychiatric population;
- clozapine obligatory monitoring and good practice guidelines;
- medication monitoring in smokers with mental illness.

2.1 INTRODUCTION

Schizophrenia usually has a chronic course though may manifest in the form of fluctuating patterns or episodes, and cognitive incapacity. This is a psychotic illness which is mainly characterised by positive symptoms including hallucinations in any sensory modality (visual, auditory, somatic, olfactory and tactile), abnormal thoughts (persecutory delusions, delusions of control and reference) and passivity phenomena (thought insertion, withdrawal, broadcast). Schizophrenia can present with mainly the first rank symptoms (positive) or negative symptoms or a mixture of the two. The negative symptoms include disorder of thought processes (thought block, neologisms, poverty of content of speech), blunted affect, poor concentration and social withdrawal. Mood symptoms such as elated mood, grandiosity, overfamiliarity, irritability, anger, inability to hold conversations, restricted range of emotional expression, mania and depressive episodes may be present in many cases. There are no diagnostic laboratory tests for schizophrenia or related psychotic presentations; instead the diagnoses rely on clinical observation, mental health assessments and self-report. Generally, the average age of onset is usually during late adolescence or early adulthood, with evidence that onset tends to occur earlier for males and later for women (Messias et al, 2007; Kirkbride et al, 2012).

Antipsychotic drugs are indicated for the treatment and management of schizophrenia as well as acute psychotic states. Most antipsychotics appear to be equally as good at controlling psychotic symptoms. Patients may react differently to these drugs, particularly with the side effects. It is difficult to predict how well a patient will respond to a drug, and to even predict whether a newer, or older, drug will be more clinically beneficial for the patient. The process of finding the right drug can often take some time, negotiation and sometimes a 'trial and error' apropoach to prescribing so as to find the best antipsychotic for a patient.

2.2 MECHANISM OF ACTION

Biochemical theories

Glutamate hypothesis

More recently, scientists have discovered that the function of the NMDA receptor (N-methyl-D-aspartate) is compromised in people with schizophrenia (Moghaddam et al, 2012). Glutamate is the most common neurotransmitter; it has many functions in the brain and nervous system. Glutamate is an excitatory neurotransmitter and upon its release from vesicles to bind with the NMDA receptors, enhances the likelihood that the neuron will generate an impulse (action potential). This increases the electrical movement among brain cells necessary for normal function and plays a vital role during early brain development. Glutamate activity in the brain may also support learning and memory functions. Any dysfunction or abnormality in production or using glutamate has been linked to many mental disorders including autism, obsessive compulsive disorder (OCD), schizophrenia and depression. The glutamate hypothesis of schizophrenia postulates that reducing glutamate levels and hypofunction at the glutamate receptor (NMDA) in the brain can result in positive and negative psychotic symptoms in healthy people and worsen these symptoms in patients with schizophrenia (Hu et al, 2015). Therefore, any drugs or agents that block the action of glutamate at the NMDA receptors (NMDA antagonists) may induce positive and negative symptoms of schizophrenia in both healthy individuals and patients with schizophrenia (Javitt, 2007). Also, decreased levels of glutamate in the cerebral spinal fluid CSF, prefrontal cortex and the hippocampus have been found in the brains of patients with schizophrenia (Gallinat et al, 2016).

Scientists have found that treatment with antipsychotic agents which block the effects of NMDA antagonists resulted in reduction of symptoms of schizophrenia (Lakhan et al, 2013). Current pharmacological investigation has focused on research around agonist agents such as 'a direct acting glycine agonist' for modulation of glutamatergic neurotransmission as a potential treatment strategy. It is conceivable to suggest that in the future we shall see newer drugs developed targeting abnormalities within the glutamate system.

A summary of glutamate hypothesis (NMDA receptor):

*   Reduced glutamate levels and hypofunction of NMDA receptors worsens psychotic symptoms.

- Drugs that are NMDA competitive antagonists induce negative and positive symptoms in healthy individuals and patients with schizophrenia.
- NMDA antagonists can worsen symptoms in patients with untreated schizophrenia.
- Treatment with antipsychotic drugs can block the effects of NMDA antagonists, eg Ketamine.

Dopamine hypothesis

Dopamine is one of the neurotransmitters in the nervous system that pass information from one neuron to another, utilising the synaptic junction (cleft) to do this. Dopamine is involved in many pathways; the most commonly talked about is related to the limbic system and the pleasure pathway, which relates to motivation, attention, thinking, addiction or lust. Found in the midbrain is the ventral tegmental area where dopamine is projected from towards the cortex and the nucleus accumbens. Increase in dopamine availability in the nucleus accumbens is associated with pleasurable activities such as sex, drug addiction, falling in love, listening to music and food consumption. The dopamine hypothesis is the oldest and most recognized of the schizophrenia theories. It has developed from clinical interpretations and received empirical authentication from antipsychotic treatment and more direct testing from imaging studies. Though clearly not adequate to explain the complexity of schizophrenia, it offers a direct relationship to clinical features and to their treatment. Van Rossum (1966) proposed the dopamine theory of schizophrenia and psychosis as being the result of over-active dopamine neurotransmission in the brain. His research provided evidence that psychotropic drugs block dopamine receptors (there are five known types) in the CNS, indicating that these drugs are effective due to their ability to reduce levels of dopamine. This theory correlates to the observations that dopaminergic pathways were stimulated by psychostimulants (cannabis, amphetamines, cocaine, crystal methamphetamine) resulting in clinical features (delusions, auditory hallucinations, paranoia, memory and mental impairment), like symptoms similar to those in people with schizophrenia. Furthermore, research has established that drugs that block/ inhibit the activity of dopamine at the presynaptic receptors (dopamine antagonists), thereby reducing the over-activity of dopamine transmission, are effective in treating the positive symptoms of schizophrenia. It is also suggested that dopamine plays an important role in the extrapyramidal motor system, with any prolonged blockade of dopamine at D2, D3 receptors (nigrostriatal pathway) by antipsychotic agents leading to extrapyramidal side effects and movement disorders.

The theory proposes that too much dopamine in the synapse within the mesolimbic pathway in the brain leads to overstimulation of receptors – abnormal processing of information, which is the basis of the positive psychiatric symptoms seen in patients with schizophrenia. The dopamine hypothesis suggests that hypofunction within the mesocortical pathway in the brain underlies the negative features of schizophrenia (such as flattening of affect, apathy, poverty of speech, anhedonia and social withdrawal) and cognitive symptoms (deficits in attention, working memory and executive functions) in schizophrenia. Brain imaging studies have suggested these symptoms may be due to changes in functioning within the prefrontal cortex (Knable et al, 1997), for optimal prefrontal cortex performance, dopamine transmission in the cerebral neocortex is vital. Thus, these observations have led to the understanding that deficit in dopamine transmission at dopamine D1 receptors might underlie the negative symptoms of schizophrenia. Decreased dopamine D1 receptors in the prefrontal cortex in schizophrenia has been reported by positron emission tomography (PET) scans. Dopamine D1 receptor which is greatly present in the prefrontal cortex is highly influential in the control of working memory, and abnormalities in working memory, which is typical feature in schizophrenia.

A summary of dopamine hypothesis (D2 receptor):

*   Dopamine is involved in many pathways in the nervous system; the most commonly known talked about is the pleasure pathway.
*   Overactivity of dopamine in the mesolimbic pathway is associated with positive symptoms of schizophrenia.
*   Hypoactivity of dopaminergic projection in the mesocortical pathway is associated with negative symptoms of schizophrenia.
*   Dopamine antagonism in the nigrostriatal pathway is associated with extrapyramidal side effects.

The blockade of dopamine on the postsynaptic cell receptors (dopamine D2 receptors) may reflect and explain the clinical benefits of antipsychotic drugs (see Figure 2.1). Dopamine receptor antagonism leads to downregulation of dopamine transmission through the postsynaptic cell. This reduces transmission of chemical messages between the firing and receiving neurons. This is the proposed basis for antipsychotic drug mechanism of action in the brain and the dopamine theory of schizophrenia. Some antipsychotic drugs interfere with the release of dopamine at the presynaptic cell; others block postsynaptic dopamine receptors and stop postsynaptic nerve cells from recognising dopamine. Almost all the antipsychotic drugs are non-selective dopamine receptor antagonists in that they block the effects of the dopamine transmission to produce no effect at a variety of dopamine receptors; examples of other drug types with similar mechanism are alpha blockers, beta blockers and calcium channel blockers. Administration of antipsychotic drugs interferes with the abnormal dopaminergic neurotransmission in the limbic system and in the cerebral cortex

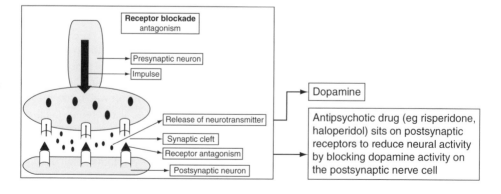

Figure 2.1 Mechanism of action (antipsychotic drugs blockade of D2 receptors)

(areas involved in the control of motivation and emotional behaviour and in facilitating organised thought) and thus can be useful in improving the positive symptoms of schizophrenia. The inhibition of dopamine transmission in other pathways, however, can result in a wide range of toxic and undesirable side effects. Antipsychotic drugs are conceptualised as typical or atypical drugs according to their propensity to produce extrapyramidal side effects (drug-induced movement disorders).

The typical drugs (older antipsychotic drugs) have a high propensity to induce extrapyramidal side effects; some of the older drugs, eg haloperidol, are highly potent and have strong affinity for D2 dopamine receptors which interferes with the modulatory role of dopamine in the brain. Interestingly, a therapeutically superior, newer antipsychotic clozapine has a low affinity for D2 receptors and induces no extrapyramidal side effects. It has been reported to have very good clinical response, even in patients who have previously shown poor response to older (typical) high-dose antipsychotic drug administration. Pilowsky et al (1993) found that clozapine had consistently low affinity to block D2 receptors ranging from 20 per cent to 60 per cent. It has been reported that extrapyramidal side effects occur only when more than 72 per cent to 80 per cent of D2 receptors are occupied by an antipsychotic (Seeman, 2014). The D2 occupancy for typical antipsychotic drugs (discussed in the next sub-section) is equivalent to and/or exceeds these percentages; this might explain the high rates of extrapyramidal effects associated with typical antipsychotic drugs compared to newer (atypical) drugs which have low D2 occupancy with the exception of risperidone which is a D2 antagonist and can induce extrapyramidal side effects at higher doses.

Typical antipsychotics (first-generation antipsychotics)

Typical antipsychotics have been available since the 1950s and are mainly used to treat schizophrenia, organic psychosis and mania. Typical antipsychotics still play a vital role in the treatment and management of schizophrenia and may offer a useful alternative to newer drugs (also known as atypical agents) when the atypical drugs are poorly tolerated. Regrettably, when typical antipsychotics are administered, they have high affinity for D2 receptors and low affinity for other receptor types. D2 blockade includes areas of the brain involved in the fine tuning of motor movement, namely the basal ganglia and cerebellum. As a result, when typical antipsychotic drugs are given to a patient, adverse effects such as motor dysfunction typical of Parkinson's disease, tremors, akinesia (a slowing of voluntary movements), spasticity, rigidity and akathisia (discomfort and a feeling of restlessness in the legs), as well as hyperprolactinaemia (increased levels of the hormone prolactin in the blood) have been reported. Tardive dyskinesia, which is a disorder causing involuntary, disruptive and repetitive body movements, is a common side effect and more evident in patients exposed to typical antipsychotic drugs than atypical drugs (Beasley et al, 1999). Although the typical antipsychotics may differ in their side effect profile according to the mode of receptor affinity, they are all similar in their mode of action and will all cause neurological adverse effects to varying degrees. The use of typical antipsychotics may also interfere with normal endocrine function and can also induce cardiovascular effects (arrhythmias), antihistaminic effects (sedation), antimuscarinic effects (constipation, dry mouth, nausea, vomiting and dyspepsia) and others (Frankle et al, 2004). The side effects of typical drugs are related primarily to their excessive blocking of dopamine pathways in the brain resulting in neuromuscular and neuroendocrine side effects (Stahl, 2008).

Drug potency is a term often used to refer to the quantity of the drug needed to yield a given effect, or it may refer to the maximum response that can be reached with a given drug. The most highly potent antipsychotic drugs come in depot preparation and are usually given in injection form. A majority of typical antipsychotic drugs are also highly potent. Highly potent drugs such as fluphenazine, haloperidol, zuclopenthixol and flupentixol are associated with the greatest incidence of extrapyramidal side effects. Risperidone, which is an atypical antipsychotic, is also highly potent.

Atypical antipsychotics (second-generation antipsychotics)

Atypical antipsychotics have been around since the early 1990s. Most second-generation antipsychotics (SGAs) have lower affinity for D2 receptors and effectively interact with other receptors such as serotonin (5-HT2A) receptors. Atypical antipsychotics target positive symptoms and are particularly effective against negative symptoms of schizophrenia (flattening of affect, apathy, poverty of speech, anhedonia and social withdrawal; Grabe et al, 1999; Pies, 2005; Holland et al, 2018). Atypical drugs are classed according to their receptor profile, ie as non-dopaminergic selective D1/D2/D3 blockers and as high ratio of affinity for 5-HT2A (serotonergic 2) to D2 (dopaminergic 2) receptors (Duncan et al, 2004; Taylor et al, 2012). Atypical antipsychotics have been shown to be particularly effective against negative symptoms and are better tolerated and safer than typical antipsychotic drugs. Atypical drugs cause fewer extrapyramidal side effects than typical antipsychotics. Most atypical drugs also act on other receptors such as serotonin (5-HT2A and 5-HT2C), dopamine (D1 and D4), histamine (H1), muscarinic (M1) and adrenergic (alpha-1 and alpha-2) receptors. This appears to be particularly true for amisulpride, clozapine, olanzapine, risperidone and quetiapine. Low affinity for D2 receptors by atypical drugs is associated with relatively low propensity for these drugs to cause extrapyramidal side effects (Abi-Dargham et al, 2005; Stahl, 2013). A meta-analysis conducted to investigate the risk of acute extrapyramidal side effects with intramuscular antipsychotics established that SGAs are associated with a significantly lower risk of acute dystonia and anticholinergic effects compared with haloperidol (Satterwaite et al, 2008). A possibly significant interactive effect of serotonin and dopamine receptor blockade is to increase prefrontal dopamine, an outcome not detected with selective dopamine or serotonin receptor antagonists administered alone (Bhui et al, 1998; Laoutidis et al, 2014). Reduced prefrontal dopamine function results in cognitive deficits seen in patients with schizophrenia. It is likely that an increase in prefrontal dopamine induced by atypical antipsychotic drug action mediates some of the modest cognitive improvements seen in patients with schizophrenia. Aripiprazole is the only atypical antipsychotic drug that reduces dopaminergic neurotransmission through D2 partial agonism and not D2 antagonism. As a partial agonist at D2 receptors, aripiprazole modulates dopaminergic transmission in both the mesolimbic and mesocortical pathway, an action which decreases and increases activity of dopamine in the mesolimbic and mesocortical pathways respectively, resulting in improvement of positive and negative symptoms (Mailman et al, 2010).

Atypical drugs are associated with a range of metabolic effects including diabetes, dyslipidaemias, sexual dysfunction and weight gain. This is partly due to complex pharmacodynamic effects of atypical antipsychotics on various receptors in the body (histamine H1, muscarinic M1, serotonin 5-HT2A, 5-HT2C and 5-HT7 receptors, and alpha-1-adrenoceptors). Clozapine, an atypical drug, is used in patients with schizophrenia or schizoaffective disorder with symptoms which have partially or fully resisted to treatment with other antipsychotic drugs, and where there are persistent suicidal or self-injurious behavioral symptoms. Due to potentially fatal idiosyncratic adverse effects related to agranulocytosis and neutropenia, clozapine requires close monitoring.

2.3 DOSE AND ADMINISTRATION

Rapid tranquillisation

Rapid tranquillisation (RT) is the process of administering medication to a person often in an emergency who is behaviourally agitated and, in some cases, exhibiting aggressive behaviour posing a risk to themselves and others (National Institute for Health and Care Excellence [NICE], 2015; Taylor et al, 2015). The purpose and aim of giving the drug is to calm the patient quickly and mitigate the risk of aggression and violence to themselves and others. RT intervention can also help to initiate long-term treatment for the underlying mental health condition. RT is a highly risky intervention in which very powerful drugs are given to the patient aimed at the reduction of agitation or aggression. Very often, physical skills in breakaway techniques and physical intervention skills are used by mental health staff when required to administer RT drugs. This is because the patient may not give consent to receiving medication in such situations and physical intervention skills are deemed necessary to ensure the safety of the patient and others. The medications used for RT tend to have a rapid onset of action, but can also have very severe adverse effects, so close monitoring of patients is necessary during and after the RT intervention. Inquiries into the deaths of patients Orville Blackwood in 1991 and David 'Rocky' Bennett in 1998 in the UK, both Afro-Caribbean males who died while in seclusion, raised some serious questions about the process of care involved during the administration of RT and post-RT aftercare by mental health staff. Concerns since then have focused on the knowledge and skills of mental health staff in providing the necessary physical health care and monitoring of distressed patients during and after exposure to RT. The findings of the inquiries also highlighted concerns of institutional bias against ethnic minorities in mental health settings, with people from the black and ethnic minority groups being more likely to be given high doses of antipsychotic medication than white patients (Nadkami et al, 2015).

As such, health providers should have in place a policy on RT, ensuring that patients who are exposed to RT receive the appropriate care and monitoring. Mental health nurses and others should familiarise themselves with local policies, as well as other related guidance such as medication management policy, physical health monitoring, depot antipsychotic guidance, injectable medicine policy and the covert administration policy.

Table 2.1 Examples of typical antipsychotic drugs

Class	Typical antipsychotic drugs	Indication	Oral dose range (mg/daily): adult	Intramuscular dose range (mg) and frequency	Intramuscular depot dose range (mg)	Intramuscular rapid tranquillisation dose range (mg)
Phenothiazine	Chlorpromazine	Schizophrenia, other psychoses, mania	25–1000 mg	n/a	n/a	25–50 every six to eight hours
	Promazine	Short-term adjunctive management of psychomotor agitation	100–200 mg four times a day 25–50 mg for elderly	n/a	n/a	n/a
	Trifluoperazine	Schizophrenia, short, psychoses, term management of anxiety states	For anxiety states 2–6 mg For schizophrenia 5 mg twice daily increased to 15 mg after one week, further increase of 5 mg every three days but no more	n/a	n/a	n/a
	Prochlorperazine	Schizophrenia	12.5 mg twice daily for seven days (75–100 mg daily)	n/a	n/a	12.5–25 mg, two to three times a day
	Perphenazine	Schizophrenia, psychoses, short term management of anxiety	For adults 4 mg three times a day, maximum 24 mg per day For elderly 1–2 mg three times a day; max 12 mg per day	n/a	n/a	n/a

	Fluphenazine decanoate (Modecate)	Schizophrenia and other psychoses	n/a	Test doses: 12.5 mg (adult), 6.25 mg (elderly) Recommended range is usually between test dose to 100 mg given every two to five weeks	n/a
Thioxanthenes	Flupentixol decanoate (Depixol)	Schizophrenia, depression	6–18 mg	Usual dose range 50 mg every four weeks and 300 mg every two weeks Some patients may require up to 400 mg weekly Other patients may be adequately maintained on 20–40 mg every two to four weeks. Test dose neuroleptic naïve patients is usually 20 mg	n/a
	Zuclopenthixol decanoate (Clopixol)	Schizophrenia, psychoses	20–150 mg	Usual dose range is 200–500 every two to four weeks but can give up to 600 mg. Max single dose is 600 mg. Test dose for neuroleptic naïve patients is usually 100 mg	n/a
	Zuclopenthixol acetate (Clopixol Acuphase)	Short term management of acute psychosis, mania	n/a	n/a	Adults: 50–150 mg Elderly: 50–100 mg (dose can be repeated after two to three days if required, maximum cumulative dose of 400 mg in two weeks)

(continued)

Table 2.1 (*Cont.*)

Class	Typical antipsychotic drugs	Indication	Oral dose range (mg/daily): adult	Intramuscular depot dose range (mg) and frequency	Intramuscular rapid tranquillisation dose range (mg)
Butyrophenones	Haloperidol	Schizophrenia, psychoses, short term management of acute psychosis, mania	2–20 mg	n/a	2–12 mg per day.
	Haloperidol decanoate (Haldol)	Schizophrenia, psychoses	n/a	50–300 mg (every four weeks)	n/a
Diphenylbutylpiperidine	Pimozide	Schizophrenia, psychoses,	Initially 1 mg daily adjusted to 2–20 mg	n/a	n/a
Benzamides	Sulpiride	Schizophrenia, psychoses	400–2400 mg	n/a	n/a
Dibenzoxazepine	Loxapine	Schizophrenia, bipolar disorder	9 mg by oral inhalation using an inhaler	n/a	n/a

Table 2.2 Examples of atypical antipsychotic drugs

Atypical antipsychotic drugs	Indication	Oral dose range (mg/daily)	Intramuscular Depot dose range (mg) and frequency	Intramuscular Rapid Tranquillisation dose range (mg)
Asenapine	Schizophrenia, mania	5–20 mg (oral dispersible)	n/a	n/a
Aripiprazole	Short term management of acute psychosis, mania	10–30 mg	400 mg (monthly)	9.75 mg, maximum three injections daily if required
Clozapine	Treatment-resistant schizophrenia	Starting dose (12.5 mg) up to (900 mg) Usual therapeutic dose range is 200–450 mg daily Total daily dose can be divided evenly with larger doses at bedtime	n/a	n/a
Iloperidone (currently unlicensed in the UK but licensed in the US)	Schizophrenia, psychoses	12–24 mg	n/a	n/a
Lurasidone	Schizophrenia, psychoses	37–148 mg	n/a	n/a
Molindone (currently unlicensed in the UK but licensed in the US)	Schizophrenia, psychosis	50–225 mg	n/a	n/a

(continued)

Table 2.2 (*Cont.*)

Atypical antipsychotic drugs	Indication	Oral dose range (mg/daily)	Intramuscular Depot dose range (mg) and frequency	Intramuscular Rapid Tranquillisation dose range (mg)
Olanzapine	Schizophrenia, mania. Short term management of acute psychosis, mania	5–20 mg	n/a	Adults: 5–10 mg Elderly: 2.5–5 mg Max 20 mg or three doses IM in 24 hours, whichever is reached first. Not to be given with IM Lorazepam
Olanzapine embonate	Maintenance in schizophrenia in patients tolerant to olanzapine by mouth	n/a	Dose is determined by current oral daily dose the patient is taking. Please consult BNF for further advice	n/a
Quetiapine	Schizophrenia, bipolar, mania	50–800 mg	n/a	n/a
Risperidone (Risperdal)	Schizophrenia, bipolar, mania	1–16 mg	25–50 mg (two weekly)	n/a
Ziprasidone (currently un licensed in UK but licensed in the US)	Schizophrenia, bipolar, mania	40–160 mg	n/a	10–20 mg (maximum 40 mg daily for up to three days)
Paliperidone	Schizophrenia, bipolar	3–12 mg	25–150 mg (monthly)	n/a

Aftercare following RT administration should include assessment of the patient's breathing (respiration), pulse, blood pressure, temperature and level of alertness. Observations should be recorded at least every 15 minutes for one hour, then every 30 minutes until the patient is ambulatory. All inpatients receiving antipsychotic medication should have a baseline ECG to rule out any underlying CVD (NICE, 2015), particularly in patients where RT and physical restraint are used often. The potential for adverse effects in the restraint process may be increased for patients receiving psychotropic or other medications and recreational drugs. In particular, serious cardiovascular effects, including sudden death, have been reported in patients taking psychotic drugs.

While there is little evidence to justify RT in mental health settings, the commonly used medications for RT purposes in mental health settings based on research data and clinical experience has centred around the use of short-acting benzodiazepines (lorazepam, midazolam) and typical antipsychotic drugs (haloperidol). More recent investigations have demonstrated the use of atypical antipsychotics (olanzapine) as being equally effective as typical antipsychotics and/or benzodiazepines, while exhibiting a relatively safer side effects profile. Note that promethazine, a sedating antihistamine, is also commonly used alongside the drugs mentioned above (BNF, 2014; Taylor et al, 2015). It is recommended that, where appropriate, psychological and behavioural approaches be tried first to de-escalate the disturbed behaviour before pharmacotherapeutic interventions are used. RT is invasive and carries added risk of harm for both the patient and treating staff. Consequently, NICE (2015) guidelines and others recommend that in all cases in the management of the agitated patient, verbal de-escalation attempts be tried first and, if unsuccessful, oral medication should be considered before any RT intervention. The option for intramuscular medication should be reserved for patients who may choose this option and/or patients who have been assessed and deemed suitable by a clinical team for RT.

Antipsychotic drugs in depot preparation

Some antipsychotic drugs come in special depot preparation and are usually given in injection form (Royal College of Psychiatrists, 2018). These are long-acting drugs which are gradually released over several weeks in the body. The side effects of the depot injections are usually the same as the oral forms; for example, zuclopenthixol (Clopixol), a common depot injection, has a high propensity to induce extrapyramidal side effects (abnormal movements). It is common practice for a small dose of depot preparation to be initially given to the patient at the start of treatment to check and assess the patient response and rule out any untoward reactions to the medication. The clinical team may choose to offer choice of depot preparation for patients who prefer this route and/or in cases in which non-adherence is suspected. The benefit of the depot preparation route is that since the injections are given between periods ranging from two to five weeks, the challenges and issues often associated with taking tablets daily are removed, and so some patients may prefer the depot preparation.

All depot medications are given via the deep intramuscular route. The most common body sites used in practice are the dorsogluteal, ventrogluteal, deltoid and vastus lateralis.

Evidence suggests that the ventrogluteal and the vastus lateralis sites are the safest to use since they are free from major blood vessels and nerves. The ventrogluteal site is preferable because it is located away from major nerves and muscles, can provide better access to muscle tissue and offers faster medication uptake. Despite potential risk for sciatic nerve injury, the dorsogluteal site is still commonly used by mental health nurses and others in mental health settings. Other potential complications associated with the intramuscular route are intramuscular haemorrhage, sterile abscess and injury to blood vessels. Depending on the size of the patient, for the ventrogluteal site, up to 2.5 mL can safely be given; for the vastus lateralis site, up to 5 mL can safely be given; for the deltoid site, up to 1 mL can be safely be given; for the dorsogluteal site, up to 4 mL can safely be given; and for the rectus femoris site, up to 5 mL can safely be given (Dougherty et al, 2015).

All depot medication should be administered using the z-tracking technique and the nurse should ensure asepsis of the body part to be used for administration and the key equipment parts (needles, injection plunger, medication pots/trays etc). While complying with full aseptic techniques and hand hygiene procedures, the nurse should observe the following steps during the z-track procedure:

- Refer to local policy to adequately prepare the skin.
- Intramuscular injections should be given into the densest part of the muscle.
- Ensure that the injection site is free from infection, skin lesions, birthmarks, scars and nerves.
- Z-track method – the skin on the injection site should be stretched and/or pulled back (downwards or laterally).
- Keep the skin stretched with heel of hand and insert needle at a 90° angle.
- Proceed to aspirate the plunger for five seconds, observing for any flashback blood in the syringe (while aspiration is still used and accepted in practice, there is no evidence to support this).
- If no blood, inject 1 mL every ten seconds.
- You should wait for ten seconds before removing the injection.
- Keep skin stretched until the needle is removed.
- Do not massage the site.
- Assess and monitor the patient thereafter.
- Document procedure.

Like most procedures involving medication administration and other clinical procedures, the nurse should take the following steps to prepare the patient beforehand:

- Reassure and promote comfort before intervention – address any fears or anxieties the patient may have about the intervention.
- Explain the reason for the intervention and gather the patient's views/feelings and/or concerns.
- Explain and describe the procedure to the patient and obtain consent from them.
- Ask and check for patient allergies and past exposure to the intervention; what are the patient's previous experiences, eg side effects?

- Check the medication chart and patient to confirm identity.
- Make sure the medication to be given has been properly stored as per manufacturer's recommendations, eg medications stored appropriately at room or fridge temperatures.
- Give medication somewhere private/quiet to maintain patient dignity and privacy.
- Wash hands and/or use gloves.
- Select the correct needle size and syringe. In practice, the 21 G size is the most common needle; 23 G size can also be used in thin patients. If in doubt, you should consult a senior member of the nursing team.

Prescribing antipsychotic drugs to smokers

Most of the enzymes involved in medicine biotransformation, a process in which metabolites of a drug are chemically transformed to a more soluble product so that they can be excreted from the body, are controlled by cytochrome P450 (CYP450) enzymes found in the liver. If the process of biotransformation fails, the patient could suffer from severe adverse effects resulting from accumulation of the drug in the body. Certain drugs, chemicals or substances (enzyme inhibitors) can reduce the rate of bio-transformation by slowing down the metabolic action of the enzymes. This can lead to increased drug plasma levels in the body; for example, significant increases in antipsychotic drug concentration (eg chlorpromazine) can occur if a potent cytochrome P450 2D6 (CYP2D6) inhibitor such as paroxetine is administered. This can enhance the effects of the antipsychotic drug as well as intensifying its side effects.

On the other hand, an enzyme inducer is a drug, chemical or substance that increases the metabolism of drugs by increasing liver enzymatic activity. The polycyclic aromatic hydrocarbons in tar (found in cigarettes) induce liver CYP450 enzyme activity and so increase the clearance of drugs from the body. As such, patients who are smokers require higher doses of prescribed drugs that are affected by this metabolism pathway, eg insulin, clozapine, olanzapine, haloperidol, fluoxetine, fluvoxamine, diazepam, heparin, warfarin, methadone, some anaesthetics and analgesics. Smoking cessation in patients taking typical antipsychotic drugs has been associated with development of extrapyramidal side effect-related symptoms due to a reduced clearance of the drugs from the body. In smokers with mental illness taking antipsychotics, the onset of extra pyramidal side effects linked to antipsychotics is less than in non-smokers, but the dose of antipsychotic drugs such as clozapine and olanzapine may need to be increased due to the increased clearance of these drugs associated with CYP1A2 induction (Action on Smoking and Health, 2018).

Similarly, the metabolism of some antipsychotic drugs is affected by intake of caffeine. Caffeine reduces CYP1A2 metabolism of clozapine modestly and can reduce the elimination of clozapine from the body. Therefore, changes in caffeine intake can change the dose requirement of clozapine.

Mental health professionals should encourage all smokers to quit and highlight the dangers of smoking to health and the benefits of quitting. Alongside this, clinicians should ensure appropriate monitoring of side effects of medications and reduce/titrate the required dose appropriately. Clinicians should strive to individualise treatment involving pharmacotherapy and provide behavioural support for smokers with severe mental illness (Mental Health Taskforce to the NHS England, 2016; Department of Health, 2017).

2.4 ADVERSE EFFECTS AND MANAGEMENT

Extrapyramidal side effects

Dopamine release in the nigrostriatal dopamine pathway moderates and keeps in check the release of acetylcholine, an excitatory neurotransmitter responsible for stimulating muscles, regulating movement and aiding in memory function. When dopamine is blocked by antipsychotic drugs, acetylcholine increases resulting in abnormal movements and motor effects. Overall, the inhibition of dopamine by dopamine antagonists is essential in the manifestation of akathisia but does not provide full explanation for the aetiology of this condition. Another theory proposed for the pathophysiology of akathisia suggests that there might also be abnormalities in other neurotransmitters such as GABA, noradrenaline and serotonin. Other drugs that inhibit the actions of dopamine to cause extrapyramidal side effects include antidepressants such as selective serotonin reuptake inhibitors (SSRIs) and tricyclic and tetracyclic antidepressants; however, extrapyramidal side effects are most commonly caused by antipsychotic medications (Mutsatsa, 2015).

Extrapyramidal side effects can manifest in various ways including dystonia, akathisia, parkinsonism and tremors, and chronic administration of antipsychotics can lead to tardive dyskinesia.

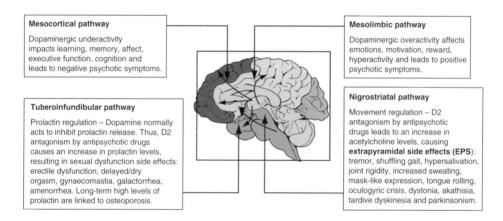

Figure 2.2 The figure shows the effects of underactivity and overactivity of dopamine neurotransmission in the mesocortical and mesolimbic pathways respectively, and the effects of D2 antagonism by antipsychotic drugs in the tuberoinfundibular and nigrostriatal pathways.

Dystonia

- Clinically manifests as involuntary contractions of the muscles serving the head, spine, laryngeal, face and neck muscles. It is very painful and often frightening for the patient.
- Usually develops within one to four hours following drug administration.
- Oculogyric crisis is a type of dystonic reaction characterised by a prolonged involuntary upward deviation of the eyes.
- High potency drugs are the most common cause of dystonic reactions in clinical settings; such drugs include haloperidol, chlorpromazine, fluphenazine, olanzapine (atypical antipsychotic).

Management of dystonia

- Stay with the patient and reassure them, emphasise to the patient that condition is temporary and that they should see improvement following anticholinergic drug administration.
- Dystonic reactions respond well to anticholinergic drugs given either intramuscularly or orally.
- Procyclidine is commonly the medication of choice (Hansen et al, 1997) and patients usually respond quickly and are symptom-free within 30 minutes. Dose can be repeated after ten minutes if needed.
- Some patients may respond well to benzodiazepines, benztropine or biperiden (Yassa and Bloom, 1990; Taylor et al, 2012).

Akathisia

- Akathisia remains one of the most prevalent and distressing antipsychotic-induced adverse effects.
- Akathisia is a term used to describe a state of unnecessary restlessness with an urgent need to move. Patients describe a state of agitation and symptom distress is lessened with movement.
- Patients complain of feelings of inner tension or restlessness, a compulsion to move their legs when sitting and inability to stand still. Patients will display movements such as shaking or rocking of the legs and trunk, pacing, marching in place, rubbing the face or moaning to relieve their discomfort (Tonda et al, 1994).
- Usually develops within five days following drug administration.
- All types of antipsychotics can cause akathisia, particularly when there is a rapid dose increase.
- SGAs such as risperidone, ziprasidone and aripiprazole are associated with higher risk than olanzapine.
- The risk associated with clozapine and quetiapine is much lower compared to other antipsychotics (Kane et al, 2009; Poyurovsky, 2010).
- Antidepressants have a lower propensity to induce akathisia.
- The risk of developing akathisia increases when more than one antipsychotic is used or when a patient is prescribed a higher dose.

- Manifestation of akathisia can often resemble psychotic agitation and should be assessed in practice, bearing in mind that other side effects (such as dystonia and tardive dyskinesia) may manifest concurrently.

Management of akathisia

- In the first instance, discontinue or temporary suspend or lower the dose of the causative agent. Normally, the condition will resolve within a week or two after stopping the drug.
- Choose a drug with less propensity to cause akathisia, eg olanzapine or quetiapine.
- Beta blocker (propranolol), a non-selective beta blocker, is a useful drug to manage drug-induced akathisia. The evidence of effectiveness of propranolol for akathisia is presented in a large scale study (Poyurovsky et al, 2006). However, patients on propranolol are at risk of developing orthostatic hypotension and bradycardia (low pulse rate); it is important to monitor the person's vital signs during administration. If results for both conditions are clinically significant, the drug must be discontinued.
- Anticholinergic agents (procyclidine, biperiden) are commonly used drugs in the management of extrapyramidal side effects. However, their clinical usefulness in akathisia remains to be established. A short-term placebo-controlled trial found no difference between intramuscular biperiden and placebo in patients with typical antipsychotic-induced akathisia (Baskak et al, 2007). Furthermore, side effects resulting from anticholinergic use, including drowsiness, dizziness, constipation, flushing, nausea, nervousness, blurred vision and dry mouth, can limit the use of these drugs in clinical settings in clinical settings. Nevertheless, patients presenting with both akathisia and parkinsonism side effects may respond to procyclidine.
- Benzodiazepines are also beneficial in the management of antipsychotic-induced akathisia, due to their anti-anxiety and sedative properties. However, the use of benzodiazepines in practice is limited due to their propensity to cause dependency and are not as clinically effective as beta-blockers in the management of akathisia.
- Low-dose mirtazapine is distinctly different to SSRIs in that it does not inhibit monoamine reuptake at the presynaptic membrane. It achieves its effects through antagonism of alpha-2, serotonin receptors (5-HT2A, 5-HT2C, 5-HT3) and H1. Histamine antagonism is associated with weight gain and sedation and patients should be closely monitored for weight gain. A small randomised placebo-controlled trial reliably established anti-akathisia properties, and the safety and tolerability of mirtazapine (Poyurovsky, 2001). Mirtazapine has no significant drug interactions, and long-term use has very rarely been associated with agranulocytosis.

Drug-induced parkinsonism

- Drug-induced parkinsonism occurs due to the action of dopamine antagonists (antipsychotics, antidepressants, domperidone) in the nigrostriatal pathway.
- It occurs in about 15 per cent of patients, and usually develops within five to 90 days following initial administration.
- Blocking dopamine activity in this pathway leads to increase in acetylcholine (cholinergic) activity, which results in the parkinsonism effects.

- Clinical presentations can be indistinguishable from Parkinson's disease. Patients display symptoms such as classic resting tremor, rigidity, slowness of movement (bradykinesia) and shuffling gait. A fine, rhythmic perioral tremor may occur (termed 'rabbit syndrome').
- Parkinsonism effects may take months to resolve after withdrawal of the causative medication.

Management of drug-induced parkinsonism

- There is a higher risk of extrapyramidal side effects in adults on typical antipsychotics and/or if patients are taking more than one antipsychotic drug. The treating team may consider tapering/reducing to a lower dose and/or discontinuing the antipsychotic drug (Haas et al, 2009).
- Quetiapine, olanzapine and clozapine have a relatively lower propensity to induce extrapyramidal side effects and the clinical team may consider changing the patient to one of these drugs.
- Lithium and SSRIs can cause tremor; valproic acid can induce parkinsonism effects. If the benefits of continued administration outweigh the risks of these medications for the patient, then tapering the doses may provide relief from the severity of symptomatology (Jamora, 2007; Koliscak, 2009).
- Anticholinergics (procylidine, trihexyphenidyl, benzotropine) and amantadine (glutamate antagonist) can be used to treat and manage symptoms. However, anticholinergics are associated with side effects including drowsiness, dizziness, and constipation, so the patient should be assessed properly during treatment.
- Propranolol, mirtazapine and clonazepam have shown clinical benefits when used to treat drug-induced akathisia and parkinsonism movement disorders (Adler et al, 1993; Silver et al, 1995).
- Provide reassurance and give the patient the opportunity to express their fears, worries and concerns.

Tardive dyskinesia

- In some patients, tardive dyskinesia develops as a result of chronic administration of antipsychotic medication.
- The term dyskinesia means 'abnormal motor movement'. Tardive dyskinesia is the term conventionally used to describe stereotypic, repetitive, abnormal movements of the face, mouth, lips and tongue, in a manner that resembles chewing, sucking or lip smacking. Involvement of the distal limbs may also occur in a repetitive pattern and has been referred to as 'piano playing fingers and toes'. Patients may also display respiratory dyskinesia, with alternating periods of hyperventilation and hypoventilation.
- Tardive dyskinesia can be blocked on request; for example dyskinesia tends to cease when patients speak or bring food to the mouth. Patients are often naive of the movements. If the patient is requested to keep the tongue at rest in the mouth, the tongue is observed to move side to side, and macroglossia (unusually large tongue) can develop. If these features are clinically significant, the patient may have problems with swallowing and speech, which could lead to communication difficulties and weight loss due to reduced calorie intake.

- Tardive dyskinesia usually develops after four to seven months of continuous psychotropic administration. The occurrence of tardive dyskinesia in patients on typical antipsychotics is three to five per cent, and special attention must be paid to the elderly as tardive dyskinesia may develop in as many as 53 per cent of patients in just under three years following drug initiation (Woerner et al, 1998). The occurrence of tardive dyskinesia is lower with atypical antipsychotic drugs in comparison with typical antipsychotic drugs. However, evidence suggests that once tardive dyskinesia develops in atypical medication-exposed patients, it is persistent for more than two years in 80 per cent of patients (Tenback et al, 2010).
- Health care professionals providing care for patients prescribed any antipsychotics are advised to remain vigilant and offer continued assessment for such idiosyncratic side effects that result from antagonism of the nigrostriatal pathway by antipsychotic drugs. Highly potent drugs such as haloperidol and some atypical antipsychotics, such as risperidone and aripiprazole, are more likely to induce tardive dyskinesia than atypical antipsychotics (newer drugs). Tardive dyskinesia symptoms can continue to manifest for longer periods (months and years) even after the drug has been discontinued.

Management of tardive dyskinesia

- As with other adverse effects related to antipsychotic use, symptom rating scales can be used in the management and assessment of symptoms. These include: (1) The abnormal involuntary movement scale – AIMS; (2) Glasgow antipsychotic side effect scale – GASS; (3) The Liverpool University neuroleptic side effect rating scale – LUNSERS. For example, the AIMS scale compromises 12 items, against which the clinician records the incidence and severity of dyskinesia symptoms. Each item is scored on a four-point scale from zero, which equates to none/absent, to four, which is equivalent to severe symptoms. Sections 11 to 14 on the AIMS scale relate to any problems the patient may have regarding their dental health and require a binary response.
- Remission is more likely when antipsychotics are promptly discontinued. If discontinuation is not possible, consider lowering the antipsychotic dosage and to reassess the patient; commonly the side effects may be due to dose-dependent effects.
- Consider switching antipsychotic to clozapine, which has been reported in open-label studies to ameliorate tardive dyskinesia (Silver et al, 1995; Spivak et al, 1997; Louza et al, 2005).
- Discontinue/taper anticholinergic medication if taken concurrently; anticholinergics may exacerbate tardive dyskinesia (Greil et al, 1984).
- Consider treatment of tardive dyskinesia with tetrabenazine (Jankovic et al, 1997; Ondo et al, 1999) or clonazepam. Clinical evidence with tetrabenazine suggests that this drug provides the highest clinical benefit for tardive dyskinesia, dystonia and akathisia symptoms, but randomised controlled trials are lacking (Chen et al, 2012).
- Vitamin E could avert deterioration of tardive dyskinesia, but there is no evidence that it improves symptoms (McGrath et al, 2011; Rana et al, 2013).

Case study 2 – Typical antipsychotic drugs and neurological effects

Background

Peter is a 40-year-old male with a diagnosis of paranoid schizophrenia admitted to an acute inpatient psychiatric ward. Peter's medication was reviewed in the MDT meeting over six weeks ago where a decision was made to discontinue Peter's oral antipsychotic medication. Peter was subsequently commenced on zuclopenthixol decanoate (Clopixol), an intramuscular antipsychotic depot preparation. Peter's care co-ordinator had reported that while in the community, Peter was usually non-adherent to oral medication; therefore a slow-release depot injection to be given intramuscularly was deemed appropriate and in Peter's best interest. Since starting on Clopixol, Peter has reported side effects including akathisia, fine tremors and dry mouth.

Management of extrapyramidal side effects

Peter's presentation is like many in secondary care where patients may become symptomatic (exhibit side effects) after taking older antipsychotic drugs and some atypical antipsychotics known to cause extrapyramidal side effects. As discussed in the preceding sub-chapters, older antipsychotic drugs have a high propensity to induce toxic central nervous side effects and movement disorders. In this case presentation, a typical care plan should consider the following interventions and actions:

- *A weekly blood pressure, pulse, weight measure to monitor for cardiovascular and weight effects related to antipsychotic drugs.*
- *An ECG to be conducted every 6–12 months to monitor cardiovascular risk related to antipsychotic drugs and/or other risk factors associated with poor physical health in people with serious mental illness.*
- *Peter's primary nurse or allocated nurse to administer a side effects rating scale, eg GASS, daily to monitor severity of existing, and screen for new, side effects associated with depot medication.*
- *The MDT (multidisciplinary team) may consider a combination therapy of anticholinergic drugs (eg procyclidine) and a short course of a benzodiazepine (lorazepam) to manage extrapyramidal side effects (tremors, akathisia) reported by Peter.*

- The nursing team should encourage Peter to drink plenty of fluids to counter dry mouth and for Peter to keep hydrated.
- The team should provide a diet rich in fibre, fruit and vegetables and provide Peter with advice to promote healthy eating.
- The MDT should assess Peter's mental state daily and offer screening for depression, anxiety and sleep issues.
- The MDT should assess Peter's response to the depot medication and avoid prescribing high-dose drug regimens unnecessarily, but if clinically needed, this must be in line with national and local prescribing formulary. All patients on higher antipsychotic drug doses must have their physical health adequately assessed and monitored.
- The MDT should assess Peter for other co-morbidities in mental illness such as anxiety, mania, depression, weight problems and any other physical health problems (Mental Health Taskforce to the NHS England, 2016).

Anticholinergic drugs

Anticholinergic drugs help to reduce the severity, and can provide relief from, extrapyramidal side effects associated with the use of antipsychotic drugs. Dopamine antagonists interfere with the modulatory function of dopamine in the nigrostriatal part of the brain responsible for movement. This leads to reduced dopamine and raised acetylcholine neurotransmission, both of which play an important role in neuro-muscular movement and regulation in this part of the brain.

Points to remember:

- Dystonia and parkinsonism symptoms usually respond quite well to anticholinergics.
- Tardive dyskinesia can be made worse by anticholinergic medications.
- Akathisia and tremors often respond poorly to anticholinergics.
- It is important to offer reassurance to the patient and assess for other medication related side effects.
- Medication reviews should be conducted regularly to provide space for both the clinician and the patient to evaluate both the benefits and new problems that may arise due to pharmacological interventions.

Non-extrapyramidal adverse effects of antipsychotic drugs

Muscarinic 1 receptor block

Muscarinic receptors, also known as cholinergic receptors, are found in the CNS and exocrine glands. Antipsychotics and other drugs including tricyclic antidepressants (TCAs) block the effects of acetylcholine, a neurotransmitter that acts upon muscarinic receptors.

Table 2.3 Examples of anticholinergic drugs

Drug	Oral dose range (mg/daily)	Common side effects	Less common side effects
Benzhexol (trihexyphenidyl)	1–15 mg Total daily dosage usually ranges between 5 and 15 mg	Dryness of the mouth Dilation of the pupils	Tachycardia Dizziness and vertigo Hallucinations
Benztropine (currently unlicensed in the UK but licensed in the US)	0.5–6 mg	Blurred vision Urinary hesitancy Constipation	Euphoria Hyperpyrexia (temperature greater than 40°C)
Biperiden (currently unlicensed in the UK but licensed in the US)	2–24 mg	Nausea and gastric upset	
Orphenadrine	150–400 mg daily in divided doses		
Procyclidine	5–30 mg		

Acetylcholine, as discussed in Chapter 1, plays a role in aiding memory function and is released by motor neurons in the nervous system to activate and/or stimulate muscles. Blocking the effects of acetylcholine by antipsychotic drugs can lead to unwanted side effects such as constipation, urinary retention, nausea and dry mouth. It is important that mental health nurses actively screen and monitor for the presence of these side effects and assess their severity through clinical discussions offered to patients daily.

Rating scales are very useful tools to screen for the presence, severity and duration of antipsychotic-related side effects in clinical practice. For example, GASS (Waddell and Taylor, 2008) can be self-administered by the patient with some guidance from the nurse. The scale has a total of 22 items which focus on the common adverse effects of antipsychotic drug use, their severity and nature of the presenting clinical features. Medication side effects can be extremely incapacitating and distressing for the patient. Often patients state side effects as reasons for non-adherence and so could explain high relapse rates in this patient group. When side effects are recognised early, steps can be taken to address the concerns raised by the patient and staff should provide reassurance, alternatives and/or further assess the patient to create a culture in practice of shared collaborative working and person-centeredness in relation to care planning.

Nurses should encourage patients to hydrate when dry mouth is reported; for blurred vision and headaches the prescriber may adjust the dose or if the risks outweigh the benefits in individual cases, the treating team should consider stopping the drug. In situations where constipation and/or weight gain is problematic, encourage healthy eating (foods rich in fibre, fruits), as well as encouraging participation in physical activity to promote health and well-being. Referrals for eye and dental checks should be considered alongside other checks discussed. Please note that chronic use of procyclidine may worsen constipation; hence, any unnecessary administration should be avoided, and always discuss the risks with the patient.

Cardiovascular effects

Generally, psychotropic medications that have a blocking effect on alpha-1 and alpha-2 adrenergic receptors, or acetylcholine (muscarinic) receptors, can induce cardiovascular symptomatology. Such drugs include typical antipsychotics, atypical antipsychotics, TCAs (tricyclic antidepressants) monoamine oxidase inhibitors (MAOI). Very severe antipsychotic-induced cardiovascular adverse effects such as VT (ventricular tachycardia) and QT prolongation, both of which are linked to sudden death, were reported when antipsychotics were first used in clinical practice. Antipsychotics can cause cardiovascular side effects such as arrhythmias and deviations in blood pressure. Occasionally, they may also cause congestive heart failure, myocarditis, further risk of QTc interval prolongation and even sudden death (cardiotoxic effects).

CVD risk is further increased in people with undiagnosed congenital QT interval prolongation taking antipsychotics. Congenital QT prolongation disorders are rare but are clinically associated with sudden death due to the potential risk of inducing cardiac arrhythmias, particularly a distinctive polymorphic ventricular tachycardia, commonly referred to as 'torsade de pointes' (TdP). The QT interval, which is the traditional time measure of ventricular contraction and relaxation represented on an electrocardiogram (ECG) heart tracing, is affected by factors such as age, gender, activity, time of day and heart rate. Thus, a more appropriate measure of QTc (QT interval with a correction for heart rate) is widely adopted to account for the effect of the heart rate.

QTc prolongation can manifest as ventricular tachycardia, which can go on to develop into potentially life-threatening arrhythmias. This can lead to ventricular fibrillation and sudden death if not addressed promptly. Other reported clinical symptoms of prolonged repolarisation in patients include fainting, seizures and sudden death. Many drugs have been found to induce QTc prolongation; patients who are given antipsychotics or other drugs associated with QTc prolongation (eg tricyclic antidepressants) are at increased risk of developing arrhythmias. The risk of cardiovascular-related morbidity and mortality is known to be increased in patients with schizophrenia. The mortality rates in this patient population due to poor physical health are stated to be two to three times higher than the general population (Buckley and Sanders, 2000; Robson and Gray, 2007).

SGAs are associated with cardiovascular side effects that can have serious consequences for patients (Enger et al, 2004; Farlow and Shamliyan, 2017). In people with severe mental illness, life expectancy is reduced by up to 25 years due to co-morbid physical conditions such as CVD, diabetes, cancers and smoking-related lung disease (Tosh et al, 2014; Scott et al, 2011). CVD and diabetes are two to three times more prevalent in severe mental illness, with CVD, smoking-related lung disease and type II diabetes being the most common cause of premature death in this patient population (De Hert et al, 2011). Cardiovascular morbidity and mortality are elevated two to three times in people with severe mental illness (Brown et al, 2010). Arguably, mental health professionals should exercise vigilance and offer screening for CVD risk factors.

- Hypertension is a major risk factor for CVDs such as myocardial infarction (heart attacks) and strokes. The atypical drugs associated with hypertension include clozapine, olanzapine and ziprasidone. Quetiapine and risperidone appear to have the lowest risk of hypertension (Khasawneh and Shankar, 2013). Assessing the patient's pre-existing condition and monitoring the patient's blood pressure and heart rate at baseline and then subsequently at regular intervals during treatment can help control and prevent further complications from arising.
- Hypotension is a major side effect observed with atypical antipsychotic drugs. Adrenergic blockade (of alpha-1 and alpha-2 receptors of arterial vessels) results in several risks, eg syncope (fainting), falls, fractures, increased angina episodes and orthostatic hypotension. Drugs that frequently induce hypotension include clozapine, quetiapine, and risperidone. Olanzapine does not block alpha adrenergic receptors and has not been linked with orthostatic hypotension, but dizziness has been reported in some patients. Ziprasidone has the least hypotensive side effects. Potential drug interactions and increased risk of hypotensive effects are seen when atypical antipsychotic drugs are used in combination with cardiovascular medications such as methyldopa, diuretics, adrenergic blockers, calcium antagonists, angiotensin-converting enzyme inhibitors, angiotensin-II receptor blockers and nitrates.
- Orthostatic hypotension is the decrease of 20 mmHg or more in systolic pressure or the decrease of 10 mmHg or more in diastolic pressure within two to three minutes of standing (Schatz et al, 1996). Orthostatic hypotension is a common side effect of atypical antipsychotics; this results from anticholinergic or alpha-1 adrenoceptor blockage. The extended effects of orthostatic hypotension have been associated with serious physical conditions such as stroke or myocardial infarction in severe cases. Orthostatic hypotension can contribute to a greater risk of injury, eg hip fractures and falls in elderly patients due to frailty and increased risk associated with a higher incidence of osteoporosis compared to the younger population. Clinicians must advise patients taking antipsychotics of side effects such as dizziness, confusion and sedation. It is recommended when assessing orthostatic blood pressure to have the patient lie in the supine position for 10 minutes, obtain baseline blood pressure and heart rate measurements, then take blood pressure and heart rate immediately after the patient arises, and then subsequently and one minute and at three minutes after standing, while also enquiring about symptoms of dizziness and light-headedness.
- Myocarditis, which is the inflammation of the heart muscle, is a rare side effect of clozapine therapy. One study found that the estimated incidence was between 0.7 per cent and 1.2 per cent of clozapine-treated patients (Haas et al, 2007). Clinical features of myocarditis are similar to congestive heart failure, and include fever, chest pain, joint pain or swelling, abnormal heart beats, fatigue, shortness of breath, fainting, low urine output, leg swelling and breathlessness on lying flat. In some cases, these symptoms may not be present. Myocarditis can be assessed from a physical exam demonstrating

irregular or abnormal heart rhythms or sounds, fluids in the lungs (pulmonary oedema) and the legs (peripheral pitting oedema). Alternative checks should include ECG, chest X-ray, echocardiogram, blood tests including white blood cell count (WBC), red blood cell count (RBC), troponin (a troponin blood test measures levels of a protein called troponin released when the heart muscle has been damaged, such as damage to the heart muscle after a heart attack) and blood cultures for infections.

- Management interventions for myocarditis involve an assessment and treatment of the underlying problem, which in this case would be to discontinue clozapine and switch the patient to an alternative antipsychotic drug. Antibiotics could be used to treat any sources of infection; steroids and anti-inflammatory medications can be used to reduce inflammation. A low-salt diet may be advised to avoid retaining water, as excess water in the body usually raises blood volume and increases blood pressure; diuretics can also be given to remove excess water. Abnormal heart rhythm may require the use of additional cardiac medications, a pacemaker or even a defibrillator. If a blood clot is present in the heart chamber, anticoagulants may be given too. To prevent complications such as heart failure, pericarditis or cardiomyopathy, treatment interventions must be initiated as soon as possible.

- While clozapine has been shown to be more effective in patients who have shown no or only partial response to other antipsychotic drugs, this drug has a 'black triangle symbol' in the BNF, indicating that this drug is subject to additional monitoring for adverse reactions, and the BNF has clear written warnings of an increased risk of fatal myocarditis with clozapine (BNF, 2018b). In their study, Kiliam et al (1999) found 23 cases (20 men, three women; mean age 36 years) of clozapine-associated cardiovascular complications: 15 were of myocarditis and eight of cardiomyopathy. Of the 23 patients, six died (five deaths from myocarditis). All deaths from myocarditis were within three weeks of starting clozapine and the eight cases of cardiomyopathy had been diagnosed within 36 months following initiation of clozapine. Consequently, clozapine therapy is associated with potentially fatal myocarditis and cardiomyopathy in patients with schizophrenia. Clozapine must be discontinued if a patient displays any sign of fatigue, dyspnoea, tachypnoea, fever, chest pain, palpitations, heart failure symptoms, arrhythmias or ECG abnormalities. Patients should be made aware of these side effects, so they can raise concerns about their treatment with their health care team.

- With the exception of aripiprazole and ziprasidone (not currently licensed in the UK), all atypical drugs (SGA) potentially raise serum triglyceride levels, and so pose negative metabolic effects on the cardiovascular system. Risk factors for CVD associated with the use of atypical antipsychotic drugs include advanced age, autonomic dysfunction, pre-existing CVD, female gender (for risk of QTc interval prolongation and torsades de pointes), electrolyte imbalances (hypokalaemia and hypomagnesemia), raised serum antipsychotic drug concentrations, genetic characteristics, lifestyle behaviours (smoking, sedentary behaviour, unhealthy eating) and mental illness (Phelan et al, 2001; Markowitz, 2008; Mwebe, 2018). Concomitant treatment with diuretics can elevate CVD risk due to their potential to induce such electrolyte abnormalities. Increased risk of arrhythmias has also been associated and linked to people with co-occurring complex needs such as drug and alcohol substance dependence. Similarly, patients with liver cirrhosis due to alcoholism and chronic hepatitis B or C are at increased risk of QTc interval prolongation and subsequent sudden death (Mimidis et al, 2003).

Healthcare professionals tasked to provide care for patients prescribed psychotropic drugs must exercise awareness of the metabolic adverse effects resulting from antipsychotic use and promptly offer monitoring interventions such as blood pressure, pulse, temperature, respiratory, weight and ECG checks in people with serious mental illness. These checks (along with others, such as blood tests) are mandatory before initiating treatment for all antipsychotic drug treatment. Nurses should promote awareness by educating patients in common adverse effects of psychotropic drug administration, as well as providing health promotion advice and screening for unhealthy lifestyle behaviours such as smoking, poor diet and sedentary behaviours (Mental Health Taskforce to the NHS England, 2016).

Weight gain and mental illness

The association between weight gain and mental health disorders is complex. There are several ideas about how the two are linked. Some scholars propose that weight gain can lead to mental health disorders; others have found people with certain diagnoses, such as depression, anxiety or phobias are prone to weight gain. Results from a systematic review of longitudinal studies point to bi-directional relations between depression and weight gain. The authors concluded that '*overweight persons had a 55 per cent increased risk of developing depression over time, while depressed persons had a 58 per cent increased risk of becoming obese*' (Luppino et al, 2010, p 225). The mean weight of adult patients with severe mental illness is significantly higher than that of the population without mental illness (Susce et al, 2005; Royal College of Psychiatrists, 2018). It has been proposed that poor mental health can lead to unhealthy lifestyle choices and increased appetite. Therefore, a combination of factors including biological vulnerabilities and increased psychosocial stress, alongside poor adherence to weight loss activities, sedentary behaviours, unhealthy diets, reduced social support and medication side effects can make it difficult for the person with mental illness to avoid weight gain (Markowitz et al, 2008; Nash, 2011).

Even with better understanding of the biochemical effects of antipsychotic drugs, the pharmacological actions underlying their association with cardiovascular and metabolic abnormalities remain unclear. The affinity of antipsychotic drugs for the H1 receptor is most closely linked to increased weight gain, though their affinity for dopamine D2 and serotonin 5-HT2C receptors might also be involved (Ballon et al, 2018). An affinity especially for the muscarinic M3 receptor correlates with an increased risk of diabetes. However, the drug receptor-binding mechanisms that underlie dyslipidaemia remain poorly understood.

Gender

The relationship between weight gain and mental health disorders has been well established through research, with some studies indicating a positive association for young women and a negative relationship for men (Allison et al, 2009; Chen et al, 2009; Luppino et al, 2010). Women appear to be more worried about weight gain than men, and hence, are two to three times more likely to pursue and be offered weight-loss treatment (Atlantis and Baker, 2008). Evidence shows that women experience more unhappiness with their weight and shape than men do and this discontent rises with increased body mass index (BMI) (Fabricatore et al, 2006). Simon et al (2006) found that the prevalence of obesity was more increased in females with a psychiatric diagnosis than in males. The study also reported that obesity was associated with an approximate 25 per cent increase in odds of mood and anxiety disorders. Various factors, including cultural, social and environmental factors, may influence the relationship between obesity and mental disorders.

Socioeconomic status and level of education

While socioeconomic status and level of education have been identified as potentially important risk factors for mental health disorders in individuals with weight gain problems, the association between obesity and socioeconomic status remains the focus of modern debate. Research has found that those of lower socioeconomic status may be more likely to experience mental health disorders such as depression, anxiety, schizophrenia as well as obesity (Royal College of Psychiatrists, 2012; World Health Organisation, 2013). A recent analysis of the Health Service Executive (HSE) database found that the negative effect of obesity on health-related quality of life was greater for people from lower socioeconomic backgrounds (The Health and Social Care Information Centre, 2013). While these and other modifiable factors may help to explain the influences on weight and/or relationships with mental disorders, the targeting of weight loss interventions in people with serious mental illness continues to face challenges, with the uptake of such interventions very low.

Age

Age is a likely moderating factor between obesity and mental illness. Younger women appear to be at increased risk of both obesity and mental illness (Atlantis and Baker, 2008; Ma and Xiao, 2010). Older adults are also at greater risk as health problems associated with aging could cause both weight gain and mental health problems. Similarly, increased exposure to mental illness or psychological trauma in older people is linked with an increased risk of obesity (Kivimaki et al, 2009; Gundersen et al, 2010).

Other contributing factors to weight gain in people with mental illness

Following the introduction of chlorpromazine in the 1950s, antipsychotics became the mainstay treatment for severe forms of mental illness, eg psychosis and schizophrenia, and affective disorders. Since the introduction of antipsychotic drugs, weight gain and various metabolic effects have been reported in psychiatric patients exposed to psychopharmacological interventions, including atypical drugs (SGAs), antidepressants, antimanic drugs and mood stabilisers. The propensity to induce weight gain and glycaemic abnormalities in psychiatric patients has been mostly linked to newer drugs (SGAs; Newcomer 2005; Morato et al, 2009; Ballon et al, 2018). Correll et al (2005) suggest the following rank order in terms of propensity to induce weight gain and development of metabolic syndrome: clozapine = olanzapine > risperidone > quetiapine > ziprasidone > aripiprazole.

The main mediating factors relating to weight gain in psychiatric population are shown below.

Obesity as a cause of mental disorders:

* Behavioural (poor dieting and binge eating).
* Biological (increased rates of chronic disease, body pain, reduced physical activity, sleep problems, medication side effects, abnormal hormonal changes).
* Psychological (poorer perceived health, low self-esteem, body image concerns).
* Social factors (including stigma related to weight gain).

Mental disorders as a cause of obesity:

* Behavioural (adoption of unhealthy lifestyles, use of food as a coping strategy, disengagement from weight-loss programs).
* Biological (medication side effects).
* Psychological (low expectations of weight-loss attempts, poor motivation).
* Social (reduced support from family and friends; National Obesity Observatory, 2011).

Weight gain in patients is associated with increased stigmatisation, social disengagement, non-adherence to medication, increased mortality and various physical health problems, eg dyslipidaemia, diabetes, polycystic ovary syndrome, hypertension, respiratory conditions and osteoarthritis, along with depression (Bray, 2004; Goff et al, 2005; Mond et al, 2009). CVD, which is the biggest killer in people with serious mental illness, is linked to the metabolic syndrome; this in turn is associated with worsening physical health outcomes in this population.

Atypical antipsychotic drugs are associated with lipid abnormalities, including elevated triglyceride levels, total cholesterol and low-density lipoprotein (LDL, bad cholesterol) and/or decreased levels of high-density lipoprotein (HDL, good cholesterol) (Lester et al, 2012; World Health Organisation, 2018). Weight gain and obesity are associated with metabolic syndrome (also known as syndrome X, dysmetabolic syndrome); a collection of conditions or risk factors for heart disease, diabetes and stroke. The clinical features of metabolic syndrome are abdominal obesity, dyslipidaemia (principally elevated serum triglycerides and low HDL cholesterol), glucose intolerance and hypertension. A common cause for all features of the metabolic syndrome appears to be insulin resistance, which can result from weight gain. Psychiatric patients are at higher risk of developing metabolic syndrome; particularly patients with a first episode of schizophrenia, patients taking antipsychotics for the first time (drug-naive), children and adolescents, and patients with co-morbid physical health complications (Correll, 2011). Ballon et al (2018) found that gains in body weight and adipose mass in olanzapine-treated subjects were associated with increased caloric intake, which unsurprisingly was further associated with development of dyslipidaemia (hypertriglyceridaemia and high total/LDL cholesterol). All of these carry a significant risk of CVD development if not properly addressed and managed in people taking antipsychotics. Unrelated to antipsychotic-induced weight and fat mass effects, olanzapine has been associated with early development of changes in glycaemic control and metabolism, suggesting that olanzapine and possibly clozapine may impair the activity of pancreatic insulin-secreting beta cells, even without the effects of weight increase (Simpson et al, 2012). Long-term exposure to olanzapine and other drugs which are prone to inducing adverse metabolic effects can potentially lead to medical conditions including increased peripheral insulin resistance and deteriorating pancreatic beta cell function, followed by glucose dysregulation and chronic hyperglycaemia. Even with this pronounced risk of developing physical health problems, psychiatric patients are often inadequately assessed for cardiovascular and metabolic risk factors (Morato et al, 2010). While considerable progress has been made in this regard, more needs to be done by health providers, commissioners, pharmaceutical industries and governments to address the obvious burden of physical health conditions in the psychiatric population.

Weight gain monitoring and management

- Assessment of metabolic risk factors associated with antipsychotic therapy should start with taking the patient's personal and family history and enquiring about type 2 diabetes, hypertension, CVD (such as myocardial infarction and stroke, including the age at onset), smoking, diet, physical activity levels and weight changes.
- Side effects of antipsychotic drugs should be evaluated at initiation, during maintenance and following cessation of antipsychotic drug administration, and measured regularly thereafter for patients with polypharmacy.
- Patients prescribed antipsychotic drugs for the first time, children and adolescents (all of whom are at an increased risk of metabolic effects) and people with substantial weight gain should be monitored very closely.
- Nurses and psychiatrists should receive training and be ready to offer advice and interventions on diet, physical activity, general health and psychoeducation to the patient and their carers. Specialist services or professionals must be sought to collaboratively assess and offer interventions on health promotion and well-being, ie dietitians, psychologists, physical activity trainers, and social prescribing should be encouraged where needed.
- All patients taking antipsychotic drugs should be offered routine blood tests before and during treatment at least once or twice in 12 months, including full blood counts (FBCs), urea and electrolytes, prolactin tests, HDL and LDL cholesterol, triglycerides, blood sugar test, HbA1c (glycated haemoglobin), thyroid function tests (TFTs), liver function tests (LFTs), fasting plasma glucose levels and fasting lipid profiles.
- Lipid profiles (serum triglycerides, total cholesterol, HDL and LDL cholesterol levels) should be specifically assessed at baseline, at six weeks and three months after initiation of antipsychotic treatment, and with annual assessments thereafter or earlier where clinically indicated. Lipid modification therapy (ie statins) should be considered if measurement of total cholesterol, HDL cholesterol, non-HDL cholesterol and triglyceride concentrations meet local guidelines or thresholds to warrant medication option.
- Patients who have multiple risk factors for diabetes (such as a family history of diabetes, BMI greater than 25 kg/m^2, central obesity, gestational diabetes or non-white ethnicity), and patients who gain more than seven per cent of their pre-treatment weight, should also have their fasting plasma glucose levels monitored at

the same intervals (ie at baseline, week six and week 12 of antipsychotic treatment), and more frequently thereafter (approximately every three to six months).

- Patients on psychotropic drugs must be weighed at least once weekly and offered a general physical health assessment. Changes in BMIs must be assessed against normal range parameters and a measure of their waist circumference to assess for abdominal/central obesity should be conducted.
- If a patient gains more than seven per cent of their pre-treatment weight or develops hyperglycaemia, hyperlipidaemia, hypertension or any other clinically significant cardiovascular or metabolic adverse effects during antipsychotic drug treatment, the clinical team should consider switching to a lower-risk drug (De Hert et al, 2009).
- Particularly for inpatients, measurements such as blood pressure, pulse, temperature and oxygen saturation should be done at baseline and at least once a week for patients taking psychotropic drugs.
- Health professionals should work with patients, their carers and other affiliated health and social care providers to assess and provide interventions to address harmful lifestyle behaviours (eg smoking, poor diet, drug and alcohol use, sedentary behaviours), as well as social and environmental determinants of poor health in the psychiatric population (poverty, housing problems, financial worries).
- Closer working partnerships should be encouraged between primary, secondary and tertiary health and social care providers to identify patients at risk and to provide opportunistic as well as timely screening and interventions.
- The simple guidance on cardiovascular health updated by Lester et al (2012) for service users, commissioners and service providers (Lester Cardiometabolic Tool) should be used alongside other strategies including national level physical health CQUINs (NHS England, 2014) and QRISK®3 to identify CVD risk and offer treatment as needed.

Endocrine adverse effects

Dopamine release in the tuberoinfundibular pathway in the brain plays a regulatory role in the secretion of prolactin hormone by the pituitary gland. Prolactin stimulates breast development and milk production in women and plays a role in sexual functioning in both men and women. Secretion of prolactin from pituitary lactotroph cells is primarily regulated by tonic inhibition by dopamine; dopamine is secreted from the median eminence of the hypothalamus into the hypophyseal portal system and transported to the anterior pituitary, where it acts on D2 dopamine receptors on lactotrophs to inhibit prolactin secretion. Antipsychotic medications are D2 receptor antagonists and can therefore raise serum prolactin levels by blocking this tonic inhibitory effect in the tuberoinfundibular pathway (Haddad and Wieck, 2004). Other conditions that can cause high prolactin levels include pregnancy, liver disease (cirrhosis), kidney disease and hypothyroidism. Other drugs such as antidepressants, H2 receptor blockers and verapamil also interfere with this intricate neuroendocrine system.

- Hyperprolactinaemia often results in side effects such as sexual dysfunction (reduced libido, delayed/dry orgasm, erectile dysfunction and impotence in men), gynaecomastia (enlargement of male breast tissue to larger than normal), galactorrhoea (inappropriate secretion of milk or a milky discharge from the breasts), amenorrhea (irregular or no menstrual periods), and long-term effects of raised prolactin has been associated with osteoporosis.

- Symptoms and complications arising from hyperprolactinaemia usually begin within days to weeks following treatment initiation and can persist during treatment, but symptoms usually resolve upon cessation of treatment.

Typical antipsychotics (first-generation antipsychotics [FGAs]) such as chlorpromazine and haloperidol raise serum prolactin severely (Kinon et al, 2003). SGAs are more variable in their effects on prolactin. These drugs vary in their affinity for the D2 receptor, rate of dissociation from the receptor and have partial agonist properties, ie the ability to act on the receptor as both a dopamine agonist (and so have the potential to lower serum prolactin) and as a dopamine antagonist (thereby increasing serum prolactin; Smith, 2003; Haddad and Wieck, 2004; Pappagallo and Silva, 2004). The relative potency of antipsychotic drugs in inducing hyperprolactinemia-related symptoms is mostly associated with older antipsychotic medication including haloperidol, chlorpromazine and older depot preparations. Newer drugs such as risperidone and amisulpride are also known offenders; olanzapine may cause mild symptoms but symptoms may worsen at higher doses. Aripiprazole, clozapine and quetiapine may cause no or little effect on prolactin serum levels at therapeutic drug doses.

It is important to discuss with patients any concerns they may have around their physical health and a psychological assessment may be appropriate in view of known adverse effects of prescribed medication on the patient's health and well-being. Health professionals do not enquire enough about sexual dysfunction, and the patient may not be comfortable or confident enough to initially raise the topic and their concerns with the health professional; however, it is necessary to seek the patient's consent, and if they agree, the health profession must offer advice and further assessment bearing in mind the sensitivity of such topics and ensure that they maintain the patient's privacy and offer respect at all times. Mental health nurses can incorporate this into the daily one-to-one reviews as part of each patient's care plan (NMC, 2008).

- Health professionals should ask patients taking antipsychotic medication about menstruation, nipple discharge, sexual functioning and pubertal development. If there are any concerns, the patient will likely require a serum prolactin test. This simple blood test to assess for the levels of prolactin can be done safely and quickly in both hospital and community settings – it is always vital to involve the patient and explain to them why this is necessary. If prolactin levels are found to be high and the patient is symptomatic, the nurse should discuss with the medical team to consider an alternative drug with a lower risk of inducing hyperprolactinaemia (quetiapine, aripiprazole) and/or lowering the dose of the medication prescribed (Anghelescu et al, 2004).
- In female patients, if prolactin is elevated above the normal range, then ask the patient if they are taking any form of hormonal contraception and offer to conduct a pregnancy test to rule out pregnancy as both of these (particularly pregnancy) can raise prolactin levels. Additionally, the medical team may consider conducting further blood tests, including serum thyroid stimulating hormone (TSH) and serum creatinine, to rule out hypothyroidism and renal failure, which can also raise prolactin levels.

In some instances, the medical team could consider prescribing dopamine agonist drugs (cabergoline, pergolide) that help to lower prolactin levels by suppressing secretion by the pituitary gland. However, dopamine agonists could worsen psychotic and manic features in patients, so patients should be well informed of the potential risks involved by the clinical team (Cavallaro et al, 2004). Alternatively, as discussed earlier, aripiprazole, a newer antipsychotic drug with partial agonist properties and also possessing lower risk of raising prolactin levels, can be considered instead (Wahl et al, 2005).

Allergic and dermatological effects

- Allergic dermatitis may occur in a small percentage of patients taking low-potency antipsychotics such as chlorpromazine; although any drug has the potential to cause an allergic rash in patients. Typical onset is between two to eight weeks after initial exposure to the drug. Patients may also report itchiness affecting the face, neck, hands and other body parts, but often palms and on their feet. The itch and rash can be treated symptomatically with antihistamines and topical steroids, but often the symptoms subside when the offending drug is withdrawn. The patient should be offered a different class of antipsychotic medication.
- Patients receiving low-potency antipsychotic medication sometimes report hypersensitivity to sunlight; this can resemble a similar reaction to severe sunburn. The patient should be advised to use sun-protective topical creams or sprays and switching to a high-potency antipsychotic is also recommended. Skin hyperpigmentation, in which patches of skin become darker, is usually harmless and is commonly associated with chronic use of chlorpromazine.
- Type 1 (immediate) hypersensitivity reaction occurs in patients who have already been sensitized to an allergen. The type 1 hypersensitivity reaction occurs minutes after exposure to the drug and signs of anaphylaxis include angioedema, urticaria, low blood pressure, rapid heart rate, swollen tongue and difficulty breathing. In 2011, the Federal Drug Authority (FDA) in the US warned prescribers about reports of type 1 hypersensitivity reactions in patients taking the antipsychotic asenapine maleate (Saphris). Mental health care professionals should be aware of the risk for hypersensitivity reactions and advise patients taking antipsychotic drugs on how to recognise the signs and symptoms of an allergic reaction.
- A rare but severe reaction that may be caused by antipsychotics is exfoliative dermatitis (also known as erythroderma) in which there is redness and peeling of the skin over large areas of the body and can be life-threatening. Associated systemic complications include: fever, tachycardia, heart failure, peripheral oedema, fluid and electrolyte imbalances. Treatment includes the use of antihistamines, topical steroids, antibiotics to treat any infection and correction of dehydration and electrolyte derangements. Exfoliative dermatitis has been reported with quetiapine, risperidone and ziprasidone.
- The US FDA in 2016 put out an alert associating olanzapine with Drug reaction with Eosinophilia and Systemic Symptoms (DRESS) as a rare but serious skin reaction.

Haematological adverse effects

Drug-induced dyscrasias (blood disorders) is of great interest in clinical pharmacotherapeutic interventions in psychiatry. These disorders may be due to drug toxicity, immunological actions or genetic errors of metabolism. Blood disorders in patients taking psychotropic drugs can include an abnormal reduction in white cell count (leukopenia); a severe and significant reduction in leukocytes (agranulocytosis); a reduction in number of neutrophils (neutropenia) and a marked decrease in blood platelet count (thrombocytopenia). In practice, agranulocytosis and neutropenia are the most clinically significant drug-induced blood disorders. Psychotropic-induced neutropenia usually manifests after one to three weeks of treatment and often is dose-dependent.

Although the risk of blood disorders is mainly associated with antipsychotics, antidepressants and benzodiazepines can also cause neutropenia and agranulocytosis. Research suggests that clozapine, an atypical antipsychotic, carries the highest risk of neutropenia and agranulocytosis, with figures of approximately three per cent and 0.8 per cent respectively among adults prescribed clozapine (Nooijen, 2011). Yet, neutropenia has also been reported when patients were treated with other atypical antipsychotics such as olanzapine, quetiapine, risperidone, and amisulpride (Duggal, 2004; Sluys et al, 2004; Cowan, 2007). Even when the risk of these drugs has been established, it is still not clear whether the risk of neutropenia is further increased when a patient is sequentially treated with different antipsychotics. Polypharmacy is common in psychiatric patients and a combination of drugs known to induce various haematological adverse drugs effects is often administered. In such cases, cessation of the offending drug(s) usually mitigates the haematological adverse effects of the drug, though post-treatment monitoring may be required for some drugs such as clozapine. However, drug-induced aplastic anaemia (complete bone marrow failure, causing global deficiency in production of all blood cell types) may not resolve even after the causative drug has been stopped.

Bone marrow suppression is perhaps the most frequent mechanism of drug-induced blood dyscrasias (Heimpel et al, 1996). Suspected offending drug agents include antibacterials, antithyroid drugs, antirheumatic drugs, diuretics, anticonvulsants (carbamazepine in particular), antimalarials and antipsychotics (notably, clozapine).

- Agranulocytosis, which is a life-threatening condition (due to the high risk of dangerous infection), usually manifests three to four weeks following initiation of the offending drug and is dose-dependent. It is more common in neuroleptic I-naive patients, the elderly and women.
- Clozapine is associated with the greatest risk of blood disorders (Voulgari et al, 2015) and is often assumed to have a cumulative incidence of 0.8 per cent per year (Alvir et al, 1993).
- Mortality from agranulocytosis can be as high as 30 per cent. Therefore, before and during treatment with clozapine, blood cell counts must be routinely and strictly monitored. Other drugs such as chlorpromazine and carbamazepine are also known to induce both neutropenia and agranulocytosis.

Obligatory monitoring for clozapine therapy

- Regular blood monitoring should be conducted due to increased risk of agranulocytosis and neutropenia.
- Before and during treatment, patients must have normal white cell count, leukocytes and neutrophils.
- Cardiac enzymes, eg troponin, should be monitored while on treatment. Myocarditis is the most publicised cardiac complication of clozapine treatment, although cardiomyopathy and pericarditis have also been reported.
- FBCs, LFTs, urea and electrolytes (U&Es) and an ECG should be conducted before initiation on clozapine.
- Baseline blood pressure and pulse measurements should be taken and observed every one to three hours during the first week of initiation.
- Monitor leukocytes and neutrophils weekly for the first 18 weeks, fortnightly up to one year and monthly thereafter.
- WBCs must be taken immediately if the patient develops a fever, flu-like symptoms, sore throat, rash, unexplained bruising, fatigue, malaise, cough or oral mucosal infections.
- Traffic light system (green, amber, red): usually used by Clozapine Patient Management Services (CPMS) for safe prescribing, administration and monitoring of patients taking clozapine. All patients taking clozapine are centrally registered on this service or a familiar service to promote safety and therapeutic use of this drug in mental health settings.

    o Green light is assigned when blood results (neutrophils, leucocytes) are within normal ranges; clozapine can continue to be taken.
    o Amber light is assigned when blood results have slightly low blood markers (neutrophil and leucocyte count); they can usually continue treatment, but with twice-weekly blood test monitoring until levels recover.
    o Red light is assigned when leucocyte or neutrophil count are dangerously low, or when there is obvious physical health symptomatology related to clozapine treatment in which case the clinical team must stop clozapine immediately. The treating team must also immediately contact the CPMS and/or other regulatory service providers.

- The amount of clozapine that can be supplied varies depending on a patient's stage of monitoring, eg if on weekly monitoring, the patient will only receive medication for up to seven days, if fortnightly, the patient will be dispensed up to 14 days of clozapine and so forth. This is done for safety reasons around management and monitoring of the haematological effects of clozapine. The clinical team will be available to review the patient on clozapine at the various intervals when the patient presents to have a blood test and when collecting their next prescription. The review can also take place during planned MDT meetings to assess overall progress and recovery.
- Clozapine assay (level of drug in blood plasma) may be performed to assess and monitor adherence to drug treatment. In cases where patients are smokers, the titration dose might have to be adjusted as smoking induces and increases the activity of liver enzymes (CYP450). The patient, therefore, may need to take a higher

dose of clozapine. When the patient stops smoking, the clinical team must assess response to treatment and act appropriately to reduce/titrate clozapine to a lower/ therapeutic dose for the patient.

- Patients who have missed clozapine doses for more than 48 hours will need to have the medicine re-titrated. If more than three days of clozapine is missed, patients' blood testing frequency may need to change.

Clozapine alert

- A patient taking clozapine will require close monitoring if:
  - systolic blood pressure is less than 100 or greater than 170, or diastolic is less than 60 or greater than 100;
  - a postural drop of more than 20 mmHg in systolic blood pressure or more than 10 mmHg in diastolic blood pressure;
  - pulse is greater than 100 bpm;
  - temperature is greater than 37.5°C or less than 35.5°C;
  - the patient develops unexplained fever, sore throat or flu-like symptoms, usually at commencement of clozapine therapy or during dose changes between intervals.
- All the above require the patient taking clozapine to be monitored closely and further assessment and tests including blood tests, blood pressure, pulse, ECG, temperature and full clinical review may need to be conducted.
- In October 2017, MHRA issued an important warning of '*potentially fatal risk of intestinal obstruction, faecal impaction and paralytic ileus*' associated with clozapine. For this reason, caution should be taken when prescribing clozapine to patients who are also receiving drugs that may cause constipation (eg anticholinergics) and in patients with a history of bowel problems or abdominal surgery. Importantly, it is essential that constipation is actively asked about, screened for, monitored and promptly treated in all patients taking clozapine.

Other adverse effects of clozapine

- Sedation, hyper-salivation, constipation, urinary incontinence (manifests within first few months).
- Hypotension, hypertension and tachycardia (first four weeks).
- Fever (first three weeks).
- Weight gain (first year of treatment).
- Seizures (can happen anytime).
- Neutropenia and agranulocytosis (first 18 weeks).

Other common side effects of antipsychotics in general include: dry mouth, drowsiness, weight gain, postural hypotension, photosensitivity, skin rashes.

*Note that antipsychotics are contraindicated in patients with CVD, a history of epilepsy and those with bone marrow disorders. In pregnant or breastfeeding women, the clinical team in consultation with the patient must always assess the potential risks and benefits on an individual basis.

Neuroleptic malignant syndrome

Neuroleptic malignant syndrome (NMS) is a life-threatening neurological disorder, most often caused by an adverse reaction to antipsychotic drugs. It has been proposed that NMS results antipsychotics block dopamine receptors which leads to muscle rigidity that contributes to impaired heat dissipation and hyperthermia (Wargo and Gupta, 2005). NMS is characterised by hyperthermia, loss of consciousness and catastrophic auto-nomic dysfunction. It is estimated that 0.5–1 per cent of patients exposed to neurolep-tics will develop this syndrome (Tse et al, 2015). The mortality rate can reach 30 per cent, and even higher with the use of typical antipsychotics. Most patients will develop the condition shortly after initial exposure; 90 per cent within two weeks of starting the neuroleptic. It can occur with any of the antipsychotic drugs, but high-potency FGAs are the most common causative agents, namely Haldol depot, oral haloperidol and trifluop-erazine (Stelazine). This reaction has also been reported in combination therapies such as clozapine and metoclopramide (drug used mostly for stomach problems, nausea and vomiting).

Physical exhaustion, dehydration, hyponatraemia (low sodium levels), young males, affec-tive disorders, thyrotoxicosis or any brain pathology are all factors that may increase the rate of NMS developing. An increased risk also occurs when Haldol depot is concurrently given with lithium. When symptoms develop, progression is rapid and usually reaches peak intensity in about 72 hours (although, this can vary widely from 45 minutes to 65 days). The duration of the symptoms can last from eight hours to 40 days (even longer with parental medication). Some cases remain mild and resolve without intervention, but in severe cases NMS can prove fatal. Without therapy mild NMS can take several weeks to resolve sponta-neously, but with aggressive treatment, improvement will be seen within 48–72 hours. With early recognition and aggressive treatment there is only a four to five per cent mortality rate and evidence suggests that mortality rates have improved greatly over the last two decades. Most patients who survive make a full recovery; however, some may be left with permanent parkinsonism, ataxia, and dementia-like symptoms (Di Venanzio et al, 2015). Early detection is particularly important to reduce mortality and morbidity.

2.5 MEDICATION ADHERENCE IN MENTAL HEALTH SETTINGS

Non-adherence to psychotic medications is very common in patients with schizophrenia, major depression, bipolar disorder and other mental health disorders. Non-adherence has a deleterious impact on the course of the illness (Mert et al, 2015). A greater pro-portion of people with serious mental illness take psychotropic medication to treat and manage the associated symptoms. Psychotropic medications are the main stay of treat-ment in psychiatry. A systematic review of 39 studies reported a mean rate of medication non-adherence in schizophrenia of 41 per cent (Lacro et al, 2002). Most patients who do not consent to treatment and are forced to take antipsychotic medication are more likely to stop taking the drugs once they are discharged back into the community. Conversely, some may be non-adherent when after taking medication, they feel provisionally better and may feel there is no ongoing need to take the medication. Also, non-adherence might be due to many patients experiencing a wide range of side effects, for example: weight gain, sedation, cardiovascular effects, allergic reactions, dermatological effects, cognitive effects and movement disorders. All these impact on the general health and well-being of patients and can further exacerbate and reinforce stigma of mental illness and social exclusion of this population from the public. Although many of these side effects may be dose-dependent, the use of high-dose antipsychotic regimens in mental health clinical settings remains common (Care Quality Commission, 2017). As a mental health professional providing care for patients on high-dose medications, it is your responsibility and role to initiate and maintain monitoring checks (ECGs, blood profiles, BMI monitoring, blood pressure, pulse, screening for neurological and metabolic effects) in this patient group; all of which are necessary requirements and mandatory. Other factors proposed for high rates of medication non-adherence include severity of mental health symptoms, concomitant misuse of drugs and alcohol, lacking insight and fractured therapeutic patient to clinician relationships (Lacro et al, 2002; Nose et al, 2003).

Generally, guidelines for the treatment and management of schizophrenia recommend that psychopharmacological relapse interventions should be considered and continued as preventative approaches for patients with schizophrenia between one and two years following the initial episode (NICE, 2018a). Arguably in practice, any consideration for continuation of treatment should be decided on an individual patient basis by evaluating the risks and benefits of the treatment with a great focus on offering prompt screening and evaluation for side effects if and when these occur. For example, in the scenario previously discussed involving Tom who had an adverse reaction to haloperidol, to promote adherence, shared decision-making must involve Tom, and the clinical team will need to record the reaction Tom suffered as a significant clinical event to inform future clinical decision-making in relation to his care and the care-planning process. Preference for an alternative antipsychotic agent, for example an atypical drug (olanzapine, quetiapine), with lower propensity to induce extrapyramidal side effects should be considered and discussed with Tom and preferably started at a lower dose to promote recovery. The shared clinical decision-making strategy between Tom and the MDT can promote dialogue and help to build Tom's confidence and trust in the MDT. Subsequently, this could improve Tom's adherence to all forms of future treatment, whether pharmacological or non-pharmacological.

Living with a complex illness such as schizophrenia often renders the person unable to maintain and sustain relationships, and many patients find it challenging to apply and hold down jobs, as well as a general lack of skills to cook, clean and budget (money management) for themselves. It is important that the MDT recognise the difficulties associated with the use of antipsychotic drugs and side effects of these drugs and the impact on the individual's life. The use of medication should always be considered as a last resort and if/when considered, this should be done alongside and/or combined with psychosocial approaches (CBT, motivational interviewing to elicit behaviour change) and regular follow-up to include monitoring for side effects and instigation of appropriate interventions/adjustments to address these side effects. Psychiatric rating scales, for example GASS monitoring, is a very useful and objective clinical tool that can be self-administered by the patient and/or facilitated by the clinician to identify occurrence and severity of side

Table 2.4 A summary of neuroleptic malignant syndrome

Neuroleptic malignant syndrome (NMS)	
Onset	Usually within three days but can be up to weeks
Symptoms	• Hyperthermia (fever, 38–41°C)
	• Muscle rigidity
	• Tremor, myoclonus (muscle jerks)
	• Confusion, stupor
	• Increased heart rate, labile blood pressure
	• Rapid breathing, shortness of breath
	• Sweating, incontinence
	• Metabolic acidosis
	• Elevated creatinine kinase, leucocytosis
	• Abnormal liver function
	*Symptoms can be mistaken for agitated behaviours in psychosis
Causative agents	• Dopamine antagonists (antipsychotics)
	• Rarely, antidepressants
Risk factors	• Patients on high-potency drugs, such as haloperidol, fluphenazine
	• Polypharmacy
	• Dose increases or reductions (particularly if abrupt)
Treatment, management	• Keep patient hydrated, comfortable and offer reassurance
	• Metabolite (electrolyte) stabilisation
	• Use of cooling blankets to reduce hyperthermia
	• Bromocriptine (dopamine agonist)
	• Benzodiazepine
	• Dantrolene sodium (muscle-relaxant) and bromocriptine (individually or combined)
	• Withdrawal of causative agent
	• Ventilatory assistance may be required
	• Monitor blood pressure, pulse, temperature
	• FBC, creatine kinase levels
	• If the antipsychotic is to be reintroduced, a waiting period of two weeks should be used for oral medication, and at least six weeks for parenteral medication (IM)
	• Generally, it would be sensible to use a different antipsychotic than the one that originally caused the syndrome.
Resolution	Days to weeks

effects. Application of such tools in practice, when appropriately used alongside strategies to mitigate and manage antipsychotic-related adverse effects, can help to promote adherence and improve patient–clinician relationships.

CHAPTER SUMMARY

Key points

- Dopamine and glutamate biochemical theories provide us with some understanding of the abnormalities in the neurotransmitter systems in relation to the symptomatic manifestation in schizophrenia.
- Most antipsychotic drugs are dopamine antagonists; this dynamic drug effect is associated with various neurological and physiological adverse effects.
- The two main groups of antipsychotic drugs used in mental health settings are the older antipsychotics (haloperidol, zuclopenthixol, fluphenazine decanoate, chlorpromazine) and the newer medications (risperidone, clozapine, olanzapine, quetiapine, aripiprazole). Sometimes the two groups are also referred to as typical or FGAs (old) and atypical or SGAs (new) drugs due to their propensity to induce extrapyramidal side effects.
- For patients exposed to antipsychotic drugs, it is imperative that thorough physiological checks including ECG, blood tests (FBC, U&Es, creatinine, LFTs, TFTs, lipid profile, prolactin levels), blood pressure, pulse, temperature and weight measures are carried out to monitor medication-related adverse effects.
- Extra attention and care should be taken when prescribing antipsychotic drugs to special groups such as the older adult, pregnant women, children and adolescents, smokers with mental illness taking antipsychotic medications, people with multiple co-morbidities and in cases of polypharmacy.

CHAPTER 2 REVIEW QUESTIONS

Now have a go at answering these questions. You might find it useful to refer to the content of the chapter to locate the correct information for each question.

1. Briefly describe the dopamine and glutamate hypothesis of schizophrenia.

2. What is the full name of the NMDA receptor and which neurotransmitter is associated with this receptor?

3. Give two predisposing factors for the incidence of weight gain in the psychiatric population.

4. Weight gain is an adverse side effect of antipsychotic drugs. True or false?

5. What is NMS and what does it stand for?

6. Give examples of extrapyramidal side effects.

7. Give an example of a high-potency antipsychotic.

8. List six best practices that need to be observed when monitoring patients taking clozapine.

9. Give clinical features that may indicate a 'red light' or worrying signs/symptoms when a patient is taking clozapine.

10. What are depot medications?

11. How do depot medications differ from oral antipsychotics?

12. What is the metabolic syndrome?

13. What clinical features must be present for metabolic syndrome to be diagnosed?

14. What are the health risks of obesity and how is weight gain related to antipsychotic drugs?

15. What are the common management/interventions for patients taking antipsychotic drugs?

16. What is the mesocortical pathway and what is its relevance to the pathophysiology of schizophrenia?

17. What is the mesolimbic pathway and what is its relevance to the pathophysiology of schizophrenia?

18. What is the tuberoinfundibular pathway and what is its relevance to the pathophysiology of schizophrenia and drug treatment?

19. What is the nigrostriatal pathway and what is its relevance to the pathophysiology of schizophrenia and drug treatment?

20. Give two examples of tools used in practice to monitor for side effects of psychotropic drugs.

21. What are some likely health implications (side effects) of dopamine antagonist drugs like haloperidol?

22. Give three examples of typical and atypical drugs and the maximum daily dose ranges.

23. What are anticholinergics and can you give two examples?

24. What is the difference between tardive dyskinesia and dystonia?

25. What is agranulocytosis? Which antipsychotic drug is mostly associated with this condition?

Drugs used in depression

CHAPTER AIMS

This chapter covers:

- the symptomatology of major depression;
- the monoamine theory of depression;
- the mechanism of action of antidepressant drugs;
- different groups and types of antidepressant drugs used in mental health settings;
- the adverse effects associated with antidepressants;
- recommended monitoring and management of drug side effects.

3.1 INTRODUCTION

The term 'depression' is often used to describe a range of low feelings, including sadness or low spirits and more severe mood problems. Symptoms include low mood, loss of interest and pleasure, reduced energy, insomnia, excessive feelings of worthlessness and guilt, hopelessness, morbid and suicidal thoughts, poor concentration, reduced appetite, anxiety, irritability and weight loss or weight gain. When these symptoms are persistent and interfere with a person's everyday life and normal functioning, they indicate the clinical presentation of depressive disorder (also known as major depression or clinical depression). As discussed in Chapter 1, the exact cause of depression, just like other mental illnesses, remains unclear but a combination of genetic vulnerability and interactive environmental factors, eg stressful life events, history of previous depressive episode, chronic poor physical health, abuse (emotional, physical, sexual), heritable personality trait of neuroticism and other factors have been implicated in the development and course of depression. Antidepressants are the first-line pharmacotherapeutic interventions in most moderate to severe depression presentations, but it is not uncommon for benzodiazepines, lithium and antipsychotic drugs to be used concomitantly. For example, in psychotic depression, antipsychotic drugs are routinely prescribed alongside antidepressants, and in treatment-resistant depression lithium (mood stabiliser) is usually used alongside antidepressants. However, in low to moderate cases, it is often recommended to offer self-help, counselling and/or psychotherapeutic interventions first before considering medication. Psychological therapies have been shown to be as equally effective as medication options and are better tolerated than the pharmacological interventions, which induce medication-related side effects. NICE guidelines (NICE, 2018b) recommend psychologies therapies, such as CBT (group or individual), behavioural therapy, interpersonal therapy, mindfulness-integrated CBT for patients with low to severe presentations of depression. Research has also shown greater efficacy when medication and psychotherapeutic interventions are used concomitantly.

3.2 MECHANISM OF ACTION

Monoamine theory of depression

Neurodevelopmental and biochemical theories propose that depression is caused by an alteration in the level or function of monoamine neurotransmitters, especially serotonin, dopamine and noradrenaline. Following the introduction and clinical reputation of SSRIs, neuro-pharmacological research has focused largely on serotoninergic pathways in depressive disorders. Neuroendocrine tests suggest that clinical symptoms seen in depressed patients are due to a reduction of serotonin in the synaptic cleft, which leads to receptor upregulation (increase in receptor numbers on the postsynaptic neuron). Treatment with antidepressants results in increased availability of serotonin within the synaptic cleft, leading to downregulation of receptors and therefore desirable improvement in the clinical features of depression. An experimental technique to deplete tryptophan (an amino acid that produces serotonin and melatonin) can reduce brain serotonin function and can induce temporary emergence of depressive symptoms in patients vulnerable to depressive illness. Low levels of serotonin are likely to occur with reduced dietary intake of the amino acid tryptophan (found in foods such as chocolate, cheese, milk, yoghurt, red meat, poultry, fish, eggs, oats, nuts and seeds). Reserpine, a monoamine antagonist that was historically given to treat high blood pressure, is now rarely used due to depression being a common side effect for this drug. Other evidence in support of the monoamine hypothesis is that the levels of serotonin metabolites measured in the CSF (cerebral spinal fluid) are significantly reduced in depression (Jenkins et al, 2016). Dopamine may also be involved in depression, and evidence proposes that there may be a collection of mood disorders in which the dopamine is altered (Barchus and Altemus, 1999). Several antidepressant drugs also have dopamine agonist actions. Antidepressants such as MAOIs (Monoamine oxidase inhibitors) inhibit the action of monoamine oxidase (MAO) enzyme found in the synapse. This enzyme normally breaks down monoamine neurotransmitters (serotonin, dopamine, noradrenaline) and, therefore, antidepressant drugs that inhibit this enzyme cause increased levels of monoamine neurotransmitters in the synaptic cleft. Hypofunction in the serotonergic neurotransmitter system has also been associated with increased violent behaviour, both towards self (suicidality) or towards others.

While SSRIs are now regarded as first-line drug treatment for major depressive disorder and other mood disorders, concerns about the effectiveness of SSRIs has resulted in the reappraisal of the role of noradrenaline and dopamine systems in affective disorders. Efficacy findings of SSRIs in depression trials consistently illustrate that a bulk of patients do not respond, have partial response or continue to experience residual symptoms on SSRIs (Nierenberg et al, 2001; BNF, 2018a). Due to these concerns, dual-acting antidepressants, such as serotonin-noradrenaline reuptake inhibitors (SNRIs) and noradrenaline-dopamine reuptake inhibitors (NDRIs), are drawing interest because of their wider pharmacotherapeutic spectrum of action. By having direct effects on more than one monoamine transmitter system, dual-acting monoaminergic drugs could embody preferred therapies for reducing residual symptoms and achieving clinical reduction (Smith et al, 2002; Thase, 2003; Mind, 2014). Significant research is being focused on the development of new antidepressant agents that modulate multiple monoaminergic pathways.

Findings from clinical investigations suggest that depressed patients have reduced cerebrospinal levels of homovanillic acid (HVA), the main metabolite of dopamine, in the CNS. Neuroimaging studies of medication-free depressed patients have also found decreased ligand binding to the dopamine transporter and increased dopamine binding potential in the caudate and putamen areas of the brain; this finding is consistent with the understanding that depressed patients have a functional deficiency of synaptic dopamine (Meyer et al, 2006).

Pharmacotherapeutic uses of antidepressants with distinct noradrenaline affinity have been subject to extensive research. Desipramine, a TCA agent with relative high selectivity for noradrenaline, has established effectiveness in the management of depressive disorders. However, it also shares drawbacks of other TCAs, and particularly has high affinity for cholinergic, histaminergic and adrenergic receptors with resulting adverse and sometimes toxic side effects. Although desipramine has generally good tolerability, it has a complicated dosing regimen, which restricts the use of this drug in clinical settings.

3.3 DOSE AND ADMINISTRATION

With many different types of antidepressants available, the prescribing of more than one drug simultaneously should only be done by specialists in mood disorders and should be considered as a last option. SSRIs are better tolerated in comparison with the older TCAs and MAOIs, and so SSRIs are usually recommended as the first-line drug of choice for depression (NICE, 2018b; Holland et al, 2018). However, a flexible approach is vital to finding the right drug for a patient, considering:

* the nature and degree of clinical symptomatology;
* safety in overdose;
* previous treatment response to a drug;
* the drug's side effects profile, interactions with concurrent drugs and physical illness;
* patient preference and clinical benefit in cases where there are associated co-morbid physical and psychiatric conditions.

As with most psychotropic drugs, starting titration at lower doses is generally recommended, and the doses are usually increased over a period of days or weeks to the

Table 3.1 Examples of antidepressants

Class	Mode of action	Indication	Examples of drugs	Oral dose range (mg/daily)
Tricyclic antidepressants (TCAs)	Increases 5-HT, DA and NA neuro-transmission by non-selective blockade of monoamine reuptake. Side effects result from high sensitivity to widespread acetylcholine, histamine, NA and 5-HT receptors	Major depressive disorder Bulimia nervosa Chronic pain syndrome Obsessive Compulsive Disorder (OCD) Panic disorder Agoraphobia Migraine prophylaxis Enuresis in children	Amitriptyline	75–200 mg
			Amoxapine (currently unlicensed in the UK but licensed in the US)	100–300 mg
			Desipramine (currently unlicensed in the UK but licensed in the US)	75–300 mg
			Doxepin	25–300 mg
			Imipramine	75–300 mg
			Nortriptyline	50–150 mg
			Trimipramine	50–300 mg
Selective serotonin reuptake inhibitors (SSRIs)	Increases 5-HT neurotransmission by blocking 5-HT reuptake	Major depressive disorder Generalised anxiety disorder (GAD) Obsessive compulsive disorder (OCD) Panic disorder Severe phobias, such as agoraphobia and social anxiety disorder Bulimia nervosa Post-traumatic stress disorder (PTSD) Premenstrual dysphoric disorder (PMDD)	Citalopram	10–40 mg (adults) 10–20 mg (for elderly and patients with poor liver function)
			Escitalopram	10–20 mg 5–10 mg (for elderly)
			Fluoxetine	20–60 mg
			Fluvoxamine	50–300 mg

Class	Mechanism	Indications	Drug	Dose
			Paroxetine	20–50 mg (adults) 20–40 mg (for elderly) For OCD max 60 mg
Tetracyclics	Enhances central noradrenergic and serotonergic activity	Major depressive disorder Sedation/hypnotic (off label) Anxiety Insomnia OCD Panic Disorder PTSD	Sertraline	50–200 mg
			Mirtazapine	15–45 mg
			Mianserin	30–90 mg
			Maprotiline (currently unlicensed in the UK but licensed in the US)	75–225 mg
Triazolopyridine	Blocks 5-HT reuptake, 5-HT2 receptors and alpha receptors	Major depressive disorder Sedation/hypnotic (off label)	Trazodone	150–600
Serotonin-noradrenaline reuptake inhibitors (SNRIs)	Increases 5-HT and NA neurotransmission by blocking both 5-HT and NA reuptake	Major depressive disorder Refractory depression Panic disorder GAD Social anxiety disorder	Venlafaxine	75–375 mg, max 225 mg for GAD
			Duloxetine	30–120 mg
An atypical antidepressant which acts on melatonin and serotonin	A melatonin receptor agonist and a selective serotonin receptor antagonist	Major depressive disorder	Agomelatine	25–50 mg
Noradrenaline reuptake inhibitors (NRIs)	Increase NA neurotransmission by blocking NA reuptake	Major depressive disorder Panic disorder (off label) Attention Deficit Hyperactivity Disorder (ADHD; off label)	Reboxetine	8–12 mg

(continued)

Table 3.1 (*Cont.*)

Class	Mode of action	Indication	Examples of drugs	Oral dose range (mg/daily)
New serotonergic antidepressant	An agonist of 5-HT1A receptor on the presynaptic neuron and an antagonist at 5-HT3, 5-HT1D, and 5-HT7 receptors	Major depressive disorder	Vortioxetine	5–20 mg
Aminoketone	NDRIs; increases NA and DA transmission by blocking reuptake at presynaptic neuron	To aid smoking cessation in combination with behavioural and counselling support. Off-label uses in UK, US Canada for depression and seasonal affective disorder	Bupropion (in the UK, bupropion is only licensed to aid smoking cessation [Campion et al 2017])	150–300 mg (adults) Maximum daily dose range for elderly is 150 mg
Monoamine oxidase inhibitors (MAOIs)	Increase 5-HT, NA and DA neurotransmission by blocking the MAO enzyme responsible for the metabolism of mono-amine neurotransmitters	Major depressive disorder Atypical depression May be useful in refrac-tory depression Panic disorder Agoraphobia PTSD Bulimia nervosa Social anxiety disorder Chronic pain syndrome	Isocarboxazid	10–60 mg
			Phenelzine	45–90 mg
			Tranylcypromine	10–30 mg
			Moclobemide	300–600 mg

optimum recommended therapeutic level. The slow titration of doses may help to reduce the incidence of side effects in the early treatment phase and hence may also promote adherence to treatment. Antidepressant effect is usually evident after two to four weeks of treatment but if no effect is evident after three weeks, a change in dose-titration or drug may be necessary (Taylor et al, 2006). Some evidence suggests that SSRIs are more likely than TCAs to be prescribed at optimum doses as titration is usually not required. In the elderly, doses should be reduced. Ideally, patients should be reviewed every one to two weeks after commencing drug treatment, including assessment of side effects, adherence, suicidality and the clinician should offer psychoeducation to promote and develop awareness around activities to encourage positive health and well-being. It is appropriate to limit a patient's access to large stockpiles of medications to reduce risk in overdose. In patients with low risk of relapse, it is advisable to treat for six to nine months and then initiate the slow withdrawal of the antidepressants; in patients with high risk of relapse, it is recommended to continue with treatment 12–24 months post-recovery. The antidepressant should be gradually tapered over four weeks after acute use, and for up to six months after long-term treatment, to minimise discontinuation reactions (nausea, vomiting, diarrhoea, sweating, headache, dizziness and tremors).

Case study 3 – Major depressive disorder and presentation

Background

Joan is a 29-year-old woman who was recently diagnosed with major depression. She is currently admitted to an inpatient acute psychiatric facility. Joan's symptoms of persistent low mood, weight gain, chronic sleep problems, suicidality and general worry started eight months ago after moving from a small village to the big city. Joan moved to the city for a better job but a few weeks into the move, Joan struggled adjusting to the hectic busy city life. Her father committed suicide when Joan was 18 years old and her mother has chronic anxiety. Joan is currently attending a CBT group as well as taking sertraline 150 mg daily, which she started about three weeks ago. Joan reports side effects including drowsiness, tiredness, feeling agitated, indigestion, nausea, diarrhoea and loss of appetite.

Effective care planning and risk management

On review of Joan's presentation, she is experiencing common side effects related to administration of sertraline, which is a commonly used antidepressant belonging to the SSRI group of antidepressants. In this case presentation, a typical care plan should consider the following interventions/actions:

- *It is usually good practice to discuss with the patient and assess the severity of the side effects, offer reassurance that many of the symptoms may stop or lessen in time, and a dose reduction could also lessen the severity of the side effects. If the patient is not able to tolerate the side effects, then switching to another antidepressant with a lower side effect profile may be required. For example, in general mirtazapine tends to have milder side effects compared to other antidepressants, and is also associated with weight gain, affecting 15 per cent of patients. This side effect of increasing appetite may be of further value in Joan's case due to her reporting a loss of appetite. Weight measures should be routinely conducted in people taking psychotropic medication.*
- *The MDT may consider short-term therapy of a sleeping tablet to help improve Joan's sleep. Alternatively, if mirtazapine is offered, this drug has been shown to aid sleep in users, preferably to be given at bedtime to avoid drowsiness in the day. Hence, Joan would benefit from the drug's antidepressant as well as hypnotic and appetite-stimulant effects.*
- *The primary nurse and allocated nurse should offer daily assessment of Joan's mental state to screen for active suicidality and response to treatment.*
- *The MDT should assess Joan for other co-morbidities in mental illness such as anxiety, mania, psychosis, weight problems and physical health problems.*
- *Health professionals should provide dietary advice, promote healthy eating and offer Joan meals rich in fibre, vegetables and fruit, and encourage Joan to drink plenty of fluids.*
- *Support Joan with activities of daily living, washing, planning and money management as necessary.*
- *Improve and promote Joan's social structure by encouraging Joan to attend community social activities and/or referral to occupational therapy for further assessment.*
- *Offer a drug and alcohol assessment. Recreation drugs can exacerbate symptoms of mental illness and/or interact with prescriptive medication. It is important for the clinician to ask about this.*

3.4 ADVERSE EFFECTS AND MANAGEMENT

Tricyclic antidepressants

TCAs act by blocking monoamine (noradrenaline, serotonin, dopamine) reuptake by pre-synaptic neurons after neuronal discharge. These drugs vary markedly in their propensity to produce side effects. Some TCAs are sedative due to histamine blockade; this is usually beneficial in patients with insomnia and agitation. However, sedating TCAs should be avoided in patients with severe psychomotor retardation or hypersomnia.

Adverse effects and management

- Sedation, dry mouth, blurred vision, weight gain, constipation, sweating, movement disorders, nightmares, increased appetite, weight gain, headache, 'hangover effect', urinary retention, sexual dysfunction and lack of orgasm in women. Depending on the severity or tolerability of the side effects by the individual, tapering the dose or switching to a different class of drug with fewer side effects is usually recommended.
- TCAs can cause postural hypotension (alpha-adrenoceptor blockade leads to dizziness and fainting), prolong QRS and QT intervals on ECG, and cause tachycardia and arrhythmias, especially if there is cardiac conduction delay. Nortriptyline, which is less likely to cause hypotension, should be considered among tricyclics and/or another drug from another class of antidepressants. People with recent myocardial infarction or congestive heart failure should not take tricyclics.
- All antidepressants can induce mania in people with bipolar disorder if they are not concurrently taking a mood stabiliser such as lithium.
- In the elderly with cognitive impairment due to dementia, confusion may be worsened if they are taking tricyclics.
- People taking tricyclics should be made aware that the sedative effects of tricyclics may be enhanced by alcohol.
- Overdose on tricyclics is very serious, often resulting in cardiac complications and is frequently lethal. If the individual is a suicide risk, having a discussion with them to limit access to medication should be considered, and the prescriber may consider giving prescriptions at intervals of days or weekly. Alternatively, other drug groups such as SSRIs that are less lethal in overdose may be preferred for the patient.
- Patients should be offered physical health examination, eg checking blood pressure, pulse, oxygen circulation, respiration, BMI measures, ECG and blood.

Selective serotonin reuptake inhibitors

- SSRIs inhibit serotonin and noradrenaline reuptake into the presynaptic neuron. SSRIs have fewer side effects than tricyclics, do not cause sedation and are much safer in overdose. SSRIs are better tolerated by older patients and are recommended as first-line treatment because SSRIs are tolerated better by patients and are associated with lower side effects profile compared to tricyclics. SSRIs should be gradually stopped to avoid occurrence of discontinuation symptoms (eg dizziness, flu like features, nausea/vomiting, fatigue, irritability, headaches, insomnia, suicide, diarrhea, shock-like sensations), which usually occur if the drug is abruptly stopped (although this is less so with fluoxetine).

- The concurrent use of SSRIs and MAOIs is not recommended in order to avoid drug to drug interactions, which can be serious and lethal. Serotonin syndrome, characterised by hyperactivity, hyperthermia, tachycardia, confusion and tremors, can occur if SSRIs are combined with a MAOI. For this reason, a drug-free window before changing from SSRI to MAOI (five weeks for fluoxetine, two weeks for other SSRIs) must be observed. Fluoxetine, fluvoxamine and paroxetine have the highest propensity for drug interactions with fluvoxamine and paroxetine the least preferred SSRIs.
- SSRIs are associated with an increased risk of bleeding, and prescribing a gastro-protective drug (eg omeprazole) to patients with a history of bleeding disorders and older patients who are taking non-steroidal anti-inflammatory drugs (NSAIDs) and/or aspirin, valproate or anticoagulants should be considered.
- Hyponatremia has been linked to all antidepressants and should be considered in all patients who develop drowsiness, confusion or convulsions while taking antidepressants.

Adverse effects and management

- Anxiety, drowsiness, insomnia, nervousness and lethargy.
- Gastrointestinal symptoms (nausea, diarrhoea, bloating).
- Weight loss and loss of appetite.
- Sexual dysfunction in both men and women.
- Tremors, sweating, headaches (less common side effects).
- Antidepressants are associated with an initial worsening of anxiety and an increase of suicidal thinking and behaviour. Monitor patient closely.
- SSRIs can increase risk of falls and osteoporotic fall in people aged over 50. Monitor patients closely and conduct blood pressure and pulse measurements if dizziness, syncope or confusion is reported or suspected.
- In 2011, the MHRA released a safety update on the use of citalopram and escitalopram at higher doses and potential risk of both drugs to cause QT-prolongation. Clinical data found that these clinical effects were dose dependent and as such, recommended daily doses for both drugs were revised to 40 mg and 20 mg maximum daily for citalopram and escitalopram respectively. Higher doses for both drugs showed a significant effect on the QT interval. Older patients, due to age-related decline in metabolic function and excretion, are significantly more at risk.

In practice, simple observation and monitoring of the patient for response and side effects is essential. If the patient cannot tolerate the side effects or lacks response, then it is usually recommended to initially trial a switch to another drug within the SSRI group, though some evidence suggests that there is no superiority in effect of one drug over the other. Like all drugs, SSRIs are associated with side effects as highlighted and the role of the mental health nurse and other mental health professionals is to evaluate daily any patients under their care who are taking regular medication. Supportive care can involve offering the patient time and space to express their fears and worries about medication side effects, and the nurse may also use the meeting to explore with the patient their current and/or future goals and how these fit in with medication adherence and concordance. Regular physical monitoring in the form of vital signs (blood pressure, pulse, temperature, respiration) should be done and offered to the patients under your care; this also meets your professional obligations and responsibilities.

Serotonin-noradrenaline reuptake inhibitors

SNRIs inhibit both serotonin and noradrenaline reuptake. Inhibition of both neurotransmitters is essential for their antidepressant action. Venlafaxine comes in two forms, tablets and prolonged release capsules. Venlafaxine has little or no anticholinergic (dry mouth, constipation, blurred vision), histaminergic (sedation) or alpha-adrenergic (palpitations, tachycardia) side effects. Older (FGA) antipsychotics, such as chlorpromazine, haloperidol or pimozide, can interact with venlafaxine and can increase the risk of dangerous arrhythmias. Co-administration of MAOIs and venlafaxine significantly increases the risk of serotonin syndrome; this is a serious potential side effect. Before starting venlafaxine, a break interval of at least two weeks should be applied after coming off any MAOI and the patient should wait for at least one week after coming off venlafaxine to start an MAOI. Taking venlafaxine alongside TCAs can increase the levels of TCAs and this can lead to increased side effects.

Venlafaxine has been associated with the development of akathisia, characterised by unpleasant and distressing inner restlessness and the need to move, often manifesting as the inability to sit or stand still. This side effect usually occurs within the first few weeks of starting venlafaxine and for patients who may develop such symptoms increasing the dose may be unhelpful.

Dose-related hypertension has been reported in some patients treated with venlafaxine. Therefore, regular blood pressure monitoring is recommended; and in patients who experience a continued increase in blood pressure while taking venlafaxine, either dose reduction or cessation should be considered if treatment risks outweigh the benefits. For patients with pre-existing hypertension, this should be controlled before commencing treatment on venlafaxine, or an alternative antidepressant should be used.

Adverse effects and management

- Nausea, dizziness, dry mouth, sweating, headaches.
- In men, sexual dysfunction, failed erection, delayed ejaculation; this can continue after drug is no longer taken.
- In women, increased or irregular bleeding, reduced sexual desire, delayed or inability to reach orgasm.
- Loss of appetite.
- Palpitations.
- Pins and needles.
- Raised blood pressure.
- Sight problems.
- Sleepiness.

Venlafaxine has a very short half-life and causes severe discontinuation problems in some people.

Examples of discontinuation symptoms

- Agitation.
- Anxiety.
- Confusion.
- Depersonalisation (feeling detached from your surroundings).
- Disturbed sleep, with strange dreams.
- Dizziness.
- Feeling of electric shocks or 'head zaps'.
- Nausea (feeling sick).
- Numbness or pins and needles.

When suspending this medication after more than one week of treatment, it is generally recommended that the dose be gradually reduced. If venlafaxine is used for six weeks or longer, the dose should be tapered over two weeks when suspending its use. Provide patients with information on side effects and encourage them not to miss any doses, nor stop the medication abruptly without clinical advice. Mental health nurses should advise patients to take medication with or after food and encourage patients to drink plenty of fluids, especially when dry mouth is reported. If dizziness is reported, patients should be encouraged to lie down and rest, and to only get up once they feel better. You should also advise patients to avoid mixing psychotropic medication with recreational drugs or alcohol and offer advice and support for health eating (eg recommending diets low in salt and high in fibre).

Tetracyclic (noradrenergic and specific serotonergic antidepressants)

Evidence from preclinical studies indicates that mirtazapine increases noradrenergic and serotonergic activity. Evidence from these studies has shown that mirtazapine acts as an antagonist at central presynaptic alpha-2 adrenergic inhibitory receptors, an action that is assumed to result in an increase in noradrenergic and serotonergic activity. Mirtazapine is a strong antagonist of 5-HT2 and 5-HT3 receptors and has no significant affinity for the 5-HT1A and 5-HT1B receptors. Mirtazapine is a potent antagonist of H1 receptors, an action that could explain its prominent sedative effects, and the side effect of weight gain linked to increasing appetite. Mirtazapine is also a moderate peripheral alpha-1 adrenergic antagonist; this action may explain the side effects of orthostatic hypotension sometimes associated with its use. It is also a moderate muscarinic receptor antagonist, which provides a rationale for the relatively low incidence of anticholinergic side effects associated with its use. Due to its strong sedative effects, mirtazapine is usually given as a single night-time dose. This is of good clinical benefit for patients with problematic insomnia who may have developed tolerance to traditional hypnotics or are poorly responsive to hypnotics.

Adverse effects and management

- Sedation, drowsiness, fatigue.
- Increased appetite, weight gain.
- Dry mouth and constipation.
- Tremor, agitation, restlessness, insomnia (less common).
- Confusion.
- Anxiety.
- Abnormal dreams.
- Drop in blood pressure that occurs when moving from a lying or sitting position, or from sitting to standing, causing dizziness or light-headedness.
- Nausea and vomiting.

Antidepressants, in general, can cause the amount of sodium in the blood to drop (hyponatraemia); this can cause symptoms such as drowsiness, confusion, muscle twitching or convulsions. Older people are particularly susceptible to this effect; the patient should be informed of these symptoms and arrangements should be made to have a blood test if the patient reports such symptoms.

The clearance of mirtazapine is reduced in older patients and in patients with moderate to severe renal or hepatic impairment. Subsequently, the prescriber should be informed that plasma mirtazapine levels may be increased in these patient groups, compared to levels observed in younger adults without renal or hepatic impairment. When switching patients to or from a MAOI, at least 14 days should elapse between discontinuation of a MAOI and commencement of therapy with mirtazapine. Similarly, at least 14 days should be allowed after stopping mirtazapine before starting a MAOI (Rickels et al, 1998). In practice, patients taking mirtazapine alone or in combination should routinely be offered physical health examinations, which should include checking weight measurements, blood pressure and pulse, as well as blood checks including glucose and lipid screening. General advice around healthy eating, keeping hydrated and avoiding mixing alcohol or other recreational drugs with mirtazapine should also be offered to patients.

Aminoketone (bupropion)

Wellbutrin is the brand name for bupropion, a type of antidepressant (aminoketone class) which also acts as a stimulant. This drug is commonly used as a smoking cessation pharmacotherapy in smoking cessation clinics (Campion et al, 2017). It is a noradrenaline and dopamine inhibitor and so increases the amount of both chemicals in the brain (Stahl, 2006). Clinical effects can usually be felt within four weeks of administration. Bupropion is associated with weight loss (Katsiki et al, 2011). It should not be used when such weight loss might be dangerous to the patient, especially when there is a history of an eating disorder that is not sufficiently managed, eg in patients with anorexia or bulimia. In the UK, bupropion is currently not licensed for the treatment and management of major depression, but it is not uncommon to find the drug used outside the terms of its licence.

When a medicine is used outside the terms of its licence, this is referred to as off-label and/or unlicensed prescribing. Prescribers take on the responsibility to appropriately and accurately prescribe unlicensed medicines, including ensuring that necessary safeguards are in place to closely monitor the patient. The decision by the prescriber to prescribe an unlicensed medicine may be based on available clinical evidence and in the best interests of the patient. As a prescriber, it is important to involve the patient in any prescribing decisions and help them to evaluate the pros and cons of the relevant clinical decision.

Adverse effects and management

- Weight loss, decreased appetite.
- Restlessness, agitation, insomnia, anxiety.
- Constipation, dry mouth, diarrhoea.
- Dizziness, nausea, vomiting, headache.
- Increased libido, skin problems.

PRECAUTIONS

Bupropion may interact with the following drugs or substances (Stahl, 2006):

- MAOIs can increase bupropion levels leading to drug toxicity; a break interval of up to 14 days is required after stopping MAOIs before commencing bupropion.
- Risk of seizures may be increased with concomitant use of alcohol.
- Marijuana, when used with bupropion, has been known to induce psychotic behaviour.
- Other antidepressants, and antipsychotics such as Clozaril, Haldol, Phenobarbital;
- TCAs may increase the risk of seizures.
- Carbamazepine may increase the effects of bupropion and increases risk of seizures.

Monoamine oxidase inhibitors

MAOIs inhibit the action of MAO enzyme, which breaks down neurotransmitters (serotonin, noradrenaline, dopamine) in the presynaptic neuron after reuptake. By blocking the actions of MAO enzyme, MAOIs help to increase serotonin, noradrenaline and dopamine neurotransmission within the neuronal intracellular structures, resulting in reduction and improvement of depressive symptoms. MAOIs are routinely used for atypical depression and when other antidepressants have been unsuccessful. They have also been found to be useful in patients where anxiety features persist. There are two subtypes of MAO enzyme and they have differing substrate specificities: MAO-A mainly breaks down serotonin and noradrenaline; whereas MAO-B breaks down dopamine. Some MAOIs are selective inhibitors; for example selegiline is a selective inhibitor of MAO-B, and is routinely used to manage the symptoms associated with parkinsonism. The MAOIs which are used to treat patients with depression are either selective inhibitors of MAO-A (also known as reversible inhibitor of MAO-A, ie moclobemide) or non-selective MAOIs (also known as irreversible MAOIs, ie isocarboxazid, phenelzine, tranylcypromine).

Precautions, side effects and management

- Dietary restrictions regarding MAOI use: normally MAO enzyme breaks down the excess of noradrenaline and tyramine (a substance found in common foods such as cheese, yeast extracts, some beers, pickled herring, broad beans, oxo, marmite, red wine); but when MAOI drugs are given, they interfere with the metabolism of both noradrenaline and tyramine. When both are inhibited, tyramine and noradrenaline can circulate at high levels in the bloodstream, which can lead to a dangerous increase in blood pressure, and can result in hypertensive crisis, stroke and can cause intracerebral haemorrhage and death. Therefore, to avoid tyramine-induced hypertensive crisis, the range of foods listed above should either be cautiously consumed or avoided during treatment on a MAOI. A persistent and throbbing headache is often a first symptom in people who may be at risk of hypertensive crisis and have consumed tyramine-rich foods concurrently with MAOIs. However, hypertension is less likely to occur with the reversible MAOIs because tyramine displaces the MAOI drug.
- Drug-free intervals are usually required when changing from MAOIs to other antidepressants or when changing from an antidepressant belonging to another group to a MAOI. Combining MAOIs and other antidepressants is not usually recommended unless under specialist secondary mental health services, eg community recovery mental health teams and/or inpatient wards.
- Potential drug interactions are very likely when MAOIs are used concurrently with other medication, and so it is important to collect a detailed medication history from the patient. The nurse should also engage the patient taking these drugs frequently to enquire about any changes in lifestyle, use of over-the-counter prescriptions, as well as any dietary changes. Patients need to be educated and advised that some medications should not be used while taking MAOIs, including some over-the-counter preparations such as cough and flu remedies and nasal sprays.
- Overdosing on MAOIs can be fatal; signs and symptoms can include: drowsiness, dizziness, faintness, irritability, hyperactivity, agitation, severe headache, hallucinations, trismus, convulsions, rapid and irregular pulse, precordial pain, hypertension, hypotension, vascular collapse, respiratory depression and coma.

Reversible inhibitor of monoamine oxidase type A

Moclobemide, which is classed as RIMA, selectively inhibits MAO-A and almost has no effect on MAO-B. This drug inhibits MAO in a reversible manner so dietary restrictions are unnecessary, though other drug interactions are still likely and therefore should be avoided. Switching from RIMAs to other antidepressants is often less problematic compared to traditional non-selective MAOIs. Clinical case studies have shown that

Moclobemide is just as effective as traditional MAOIs and so this drug has become more routinely used in practice (Youdim et al, 2006).

Side effects

* Weight gain.
* Dry mouth.
* Nausea.
* Postural hypotension.
* Skin reactions.
* Dizziness.
* Low blood pressure.
* Involuntary muscle jerks or muscle aches.
* Reduced sexual desire or decreased sexual ability.
* Difficulty urinating.
* Diarrhoea or constipation.
* Drowsiness.
* Headache and palpitations.
* Insomnia or other sleep disturbance.
* Agitation.

Serotonin syndrome

Serotonin syndrome is a term used to refer to a cluster of motor, autonomic and mental changes resulting from excess serotonin neurotransmission. Serotonin syndrome can occur when medications that cause high levels of serotonin to accumulate in the body are administered. It often occurs either during dose changes or when adding new drugs. Some illegal drugs and dietary supplements are also associated with serotonin syndrome. Symptoms can range from mild (shivering and diarrhoea) to severe (muscle rigidity, fever, seizures, confusion, rapid heart rate, high blood pressure, dilated pupils, loss of muscle co-ordination or twitching muscles). Severe serotonin syndrome can be fatal if not treated. Symptom onset is usually rapid and can occur within minutes; mental health nurses must exercise vigilance and be aware of the symptoms described above to be able to quickly identify any cases in which elevated serotonin levels are suspected and thus promptly trigger the necessary clinical response.

Drugs implicated in serotonin syndrome include SSRIs, SNRIs, TCAs, MAOIs, St John's Wort and lithium. The risks of serotonin syndrome when taking either a SSRI or SNRI in combination with tramadol are very serious and can be fatal if not urgently managed. Other drugs that have been reported and can elevate serotonin levels include pethidine, fentanyl, dextromethorphan and recreational drugs, eg cocaine, MDMA (methylenedioxymethamphetamine) and amphetamine. When prescribing, it is always worth checking whether there are any known drug interactions likely to cause serotonin syndrome and assess the clinical benefits of the proposed intervention against the risks. It is generally not recommended to use more than one antidepressant concomitantly as this further increases the risk of developing serotonin syndrome.

Management of serotonin syndrome initially involves discontinuing the causative agents first. Benzodiazepines are the first line of therapy to treat hyperreflexia, agitation, tremors and muscle rigidity. Generally, in all suspected cases, careful observation of the patient is advised, particularly during treatment initiation, dose increases and changes; and seek senior help immediately if you are concerned about the patient. Patients who present with moderate to severe serotonin syndrome may require hospitalisation and patients with hyperthermia (a temperature greater than 41.1°C) who are critically ill may often require neuromuscular paralysis and tracheal intubation. Timely screening and supportive care given early could reduce further complications and may provide a more favourable prognosis.

To offer continued management for adverse effects related to pharmacological interventions and/or signs resulting from poor physical health, the mental health nurse and/or mental health professionals should use the National Early Warning Score (NEWS 2) to promptly screen and assess patients at risk of further deterioration and seek urgent medical advice where appropriate. The NEWS score is a simple tool based on an aggregate scoring where a score is given to each of the six physiological parameters/measurements (Royal College of Physicians, 2018).

3.5 DIFFERENCES IN THERAPEUTIC EFFECTS OF ANTIDEPRESSANTS

Initial treatment with antidepressants may be beneficial in 50 to 60 per cent of patients with true antidepressant effect usually taking weeks for symptoms to improve (Frodl, 2017). This commonly complicates treatment and can result in increased risk of suicidal behaviour. Partly, this is due to lack of understanding of the exact biological mechanisms of depression and the precise mechanism of action of current pharmacological interventions. A large multi-centre study found that a few of the patients with major depressive disorder attained remission within 10–14 weeks of starting treatment (Trivedi et al, 2006). Similarly, another study of outpatients with major depressive disorder who received a sufficient initial pharmacotherapeutic intervention in the form of a first-line treatment (SSRI) reported that only 29–46 per cent were recorded as having adequately responded (Fava, 2000). Alarmingly, the delayed onset of antidepressant action is linked to serious negative effects; a study into antidepressant action and suicidality found an increased risk of suicidal behaviour during the first month of treatment with antidepressants, particularly in the first nine days. This risk was similar irrespective of the class of antidepressant, eg amitriptyline, fluoxetine, paroxetine or dothiepin (Jick et al, 2004). It is also thought that the reason for increased suicidal risk may be due to increased energy and motivation in patients due to raised noradrenaline and dopamine in patients at the beginning of the treatment, but that low mood takes longer to lift and that during this interim period the patient still has low mood and negative thoughts but increased energy levels and motivation which can worsen and trigger increased risk of suicidality. Therefore, mental health professionals caring for patients starting antidepressants or having dose changes must monitor the high risk of suicidal behaviour and/or other deliberate self-harm during the first month of treatment. Similarly, delayed onset of antidepressant mechanism of action could be related to psychosocial stressors and complex, environmental factors which may exacerbate depression and impact on quality of life by impairing the patient's ability to function socially and occupationally.

In general, TCAs are thought to have superior antidepressant effectiveness, but they have been largely replaced by the SSRIs which are almost as equally effective, are better tolerated, have limited side effects, are less toxic in overdose and provide ease of dosing (Thase, 2003; Duncan et al, 2004). Evidence indicates that SSRIs are often an inadequate treatment for more severe depressive illness. Moreover, MAOIs and TCAs have direct pharmacological actions on more than one monoamine neurotransmitter system, and both classes of antidepressants are reputed to have superior clinical efficacy and may be more effective in severe depression (Thase et al, 1995; Robinson, 2002; Duncan et al, 2004). However, at higher doses some of the newer drugs, for example citalopram, can definitely be more toxic than some older drugs, and evidence that some old drugs are more effective than some of the new drugs remains strong, especially for amitriptyline and clomipramine. The recognised effectiveness of these FGAs (first generation antidepressants) has prompted development and research into newer dual-acting antidepressants with superior receptor specificity (eg SNRIs venlafaxine and duloxetine). In comparative clinical trials, these agents have shown equal if not superior effectiveness to SSRIs (Nemeroff et al, 2002; Smith et al, 2002; Krüger, 2007).

Antidepressants have a prompt onset of action and non-response at 2–6 weeks is a good predictor of overall response. If the patient reports some improvement during this time, continue and assess for a further 2–3 weeks and offer ongoing reviews as appropriate. The absence of any improvement at all at 3–4 weeks should normally provoke a change in treatment, response failure to an antidepressant does not predict response to another drug class or another drug within a class. All antidepressants are associated with initial worsening of anxiety or agitation and an increase of suicidal thinking and behaviour. Also, prescribers should withdraw antidepressants gradually and always inform patients of the risk and nature of discontinuation symptoms (these were discussed in the sub-section on venlafaxine).

CHAPTER SUMMARY

Key points

- The monoamine theory of depression implicates abnormalities in monoamine neurotransmitter systems, eg dopamine, serotonin, noradrenaline.
- There are various classes of antidepressants. The older groups of drugs are the TCAs and MAOI. The newer drugs include SSRIs, SNRIs, mirtazapine and bupropion.

- Just like antipsychotic medications, antidepressants are associated with a diverse range and degree of physiological and neurological adverse effects.
- Patients should be reviewed every one to two weeks after commencing antidepressants, including assessment of side effects, adherence and suicidality (which may be induced by the medication as some drugs such as fluoxetine have been reported to escalate suicidal tendencies in the depressed clients; young people are most at risk). The clinician should offer psychoeducation to develop awareness around activities to promote mental health and well-being.
- Physical health monitoring of metabolic effects and other parameters in the depressed patient taking antidepressants and other drugs should include interventions such as: ECG, blood tests (FBC, U&Es, creatinine, LFTs, TFT, lipids), blood pressure, pulse, temperature, weight/BMI measures (Mental Health Taskforce to the NHS England, 2016).

CHAPTER 3 REVIEW QUESTIONS

Now have a go at answering these questions. You might find it useful to refer to the content of the chapter to locate the correct information for each question.

1. What is the general mechanism of action of antidepressants?

2. What is serotonin and why is it relevant to the monoamine theory of depression?

3. What is your understanding of the term clinical depression?

4. What class of drug does amitriptyline belong to? State its clinical uses.

5. What is serotonin syndrome, and can you describe the symptoms?

6. What is the usual dose range of citalopram and why is it not recommended over doses greater than 40 mg?

7. Suicidal thoughts are a potential side effect of antidepressants. True or false?

8. What is St John's Wort?

9. What does SSRI stand for? Give three examples of drugs from this class.

10. What is tyramine and why is this chemical relevant to patients taking MAOIs?

11. When switching from a SSRI to MAOI, how many days should elapse before starting MAOIs?

12. List some of the common side effects of SSRIs.

13. What factors should prescribers consider in selection and/or choice of an antidepressant?

14. What cardiovascular adverse effects are associated with TCAs?

15. Which class of antidepressants is recommended by NICE as a first choice for treatment of moderate to severe major depressive disorder?

16. Name some of the common foods rich in tyramine.

17. What signs/symptoms may occur if antidepressants are withdrawn abruptly?

18. What are the clinical indications of bupropion?

19. What physical health measures might you need to carry out to monitor a patient taking antidepressants?

20. All antidepressants can induce_____in people with bipolar disorder if they are not concurrently taking a mood stabiliser such as lithium. Fill in the missing words.

4 Drugs used in dementia

CHAPTER AIMS

This chapter covers:

- the symptomatology of dementia;
- the mechanism of action of anti-dementia drugs;
- different groups and types of anti-dementia drugs used in mental health settings;
- the adverse effects associated with anti-dementia drugs;
- recommended monitoring and management of drug side effects;
- polypharmacy and the care of older patients.

4.1 INTRODUCTION

Neuro-degeneration and structural damage to brain cells of higher cortical function presents clinical symptoms such as decline in memory, thinking, comprehension, orientation, language, personality, intellect and behaviour. Other commonly reported symptoms of dementia include behavioural changes, language and communication difficulties, aggression and hallucinations. The amyloid cascade theory has been proposed to explain the aetiology of Alzheimer's disease. The theory proposes that over-activity and accumulation of large proteins (amyloid beta) that are toxic to brain cells result in the degeneration of brain cells and subsequently Alzheimer's disease. The organic disease of the subcortical structures is usually, but not necessarily, progressive and irreversible. Anti-dementia drugs, also known as cognitive enhancers, are routinely used for the management of cognitive symptoms in Alzheimer's disease (the most common type of dementia) and other dementias including vascular dementia, lewy body dementia, frontotemporal. Anti-dementia drugs can temporarily alleviate symptoms, or slow down the progress of symptoms of dementia in some patients. There are currently no drugs that can provide a cure for Alzheimer's disease or other types of dementia. Antidepressants or antipsychotics may be used to manage behavioural and psychological symptoms associated with dementia such as agitation, delusions, depression and aggression – these may also be improved by cognitive enhancers (Farlow et al, 2007; Taylor et al, 2012). Symptoms of dementia may be caused by several conditions. Therefore, medical and psychological co-morbidities should be investigated and treated, including physical illness (dehydration, infections, malnutrition, anaemia, psychiatric illness, hypothermia, depression and any sensory impairment).

4.2 MECHANISM OF ACTION

Acetylcholinesterase inhibitors

Biochemical abnormalities of acetylcholine in the basal forebrain (cerebral cortex and hippocampus) have been implicated in the aetiology and pathology of Alzheimer's disease. Acetylcholine is an excitatory neurotransmitter with roles in memory function and stimulates fine muscle movement. Effects of reduced acetylcholine can result in poor memory, poor concentration, euphoria, lack of inhibition, antisocial behaviour, manic behaviour and speech problems. Drug interventions in Alzheimer's disease, such as acetylcholinesterase inhibitors, act to inhibit breakdown of acetylcholine by the enzyme acetylcholinesterase. This results in increased neurotransmission of acetylcholine – thereby enhancing cognitive function. Acetylcholinesterase inhibitors, such as donepezil, galantamine and rivastigmine, block or reduce the activity of acetylcholinesterase and so increase acetylcholine transmission leading to increased communication between nerve cells, which in turn may temporarily improve, stabilise or slow the worsening of symptoms of dementia.

The effect of the drugs varies widely for different people. Some may not notice any effect; others may find their symptoms improve slightly. Patients may find the drugs help to slow the progression of the disease; hence their symptoms become gradually worse over time, rather than the faster deterioration they noticed prior to drug treatment. Patients that have been prescribed acetylcholinesterase inhibitors should be reviewed within a month of starting the drug and again within six months to assess quality of life, cognitive function and behavioural symptoms. There is no way to predict how an individual will respond. The aspects in which some people with Alzheimer's disease may find improvement are:

- ability to think clearly and motivation;
- reduced anxiety;
- memory;
- function in daily activities, eg personal care, shopping and dressing;
- behavioural and psychological symptoms.

Acetylcholinesterase (cholinesterase) inhibitors treat the symptoms of Alzheimer's disease only and are not a cure – there is no evidence that these drugs can stop or reverse the process of nerve cell loss that causes Alzheimer's disease. It is crucial to emphasise that the drugs may not help all patients prescribed these medications and that the individual's response cannot be predicted. All cholinesterase inhibitors work in a similar way; however, one might suit an individual better than another, especially in relation to side effects and tolerability. Results from clinical trials indicate that cholinesterase inhibitors may provide limited benefits for people with mild to moderately severe Alzheimer's disease and for people with dementia with Lewy bodies, vascular dementia or mixed dementia (McKeith et al, 2000; Emre et al, 2004).

The guidance from NICE (2016) recommends that donepezil, rivastigmine or galantamine is offered as part of NHS care for people with mild to moderate Alzheimer's disease. There is good evidence (strongest for donepezil) that cholinesterase inhibitors help
people with more severe Alzheimer's disease (Feldman et al, 2011). Between 40–70 per
cent of people with Alzheimer's disease benefit from taking a cholinesterase inhibitor
(Bullock et al, 2005). In cases with treatment benefit, symptoms tend to improve temporarily (for between 6 and 12 months in most cases) and may then gradually worsen over
the following months.

4.3 DOSE AND ADMINISTRATION

Table 4.1 Examples of anti-dementia drugs

Class	Indication	Examples of drugs	Oral dose range (mg/daily)
acetylcholinesterase inhibitors	Alzheimer's disease Dementia with Lewy bodies Dementia in Parkinson's disease Mixed dementias (Alzheimer's disease and vascular dementia)	Donepezil	5 mg once daily in the evening for one month, review and if required, increase to 10 mg daily.
		Rivastigmine	3–12 mg (capsules) Rivastigmine daily patches are also available. These deliver daily doses of 4.6 mg, 9.5 mg or 13.3 mg, with fewer side effects than the capsules. Patches are suited to patients who may struggle with taking medication by mouth; they are popular with carers. Only one patch should be applied at any one time and it should be put on different parts of the skin each time, to avoid causing a rash.

(*continued*)

Table 4.1 (*Cont.*)

Class	Indication	Examples of drugs	Oral dose range (mg/daily)
		Galantamine	The recommended starting dose for galantamine is 8 mg daily for four weeks, increasing to 16 mg a day for another four weeks. Usual daily dose range is 16–24 mg. Galantamine is made in a variety of forms including a 4 mg/ml (twice daily) oral solution, and tablets of 8 mg and 12 mg. Slow-release (XL) capsules are available in doses of 8 mg, 16 mg and 24 mg; these are popular because they only need to be taken once a day.
NMDA receptor antagonist	Moderate-to-severe Alzheimer's disease. For patients with moderate dementia who cannot take the cholinesterase inhibitor drugs. In patients in the middle-later stages of the disease, it can slow down the progression of symptoms, including disorientation and difficulties	Memantine	Recommended starting dose is 5 mg daily, increased by 5 mg weekly, up to maximum of 20 mg a day after four weeks. Memantine comes in two forms: as 10 mg and 20 mg tablets, and as 10 mg oral drops. The 10 mg tablets can be broken in half (into 5 mg doses) and taken with or without food.

Table 4.1 (*Cont.*)

Class	Indication	Examples of drugs	Oral dose range (mg/daily)
	carrying out daily activities. Memantine has also shown effectiveness against symptoms including delusions, aggression and agitation.		

4.4 ADVERSE EFFECTS AND MANAGEMENT

Acetylcholinesterase inhibitors

Acetylcholinesterase inhibitors are well tolerated and safe. Contraindications include presence of significant electrocardiographic abnormalities, peptic ulcer disease and significant chronic obstructive pulmonary disease. Adverse events are more common at commencement of treatment and at dose increase; these are mostly gastrointestinal – nausea, vomiting or diarrhoea, which often respond to symptomatic treatment. Symptomatic bradycardia and syncope can occur but are rare (Hernandez et al, 2009). In one study the five most common side effects were, in order of frequency of presentation: nausea, agitation, vomiting, headache and fainting. In the long term, the most frequent side effects from cholinesterase inhibitors are: muscle cramps, tremors, nightmares, nausea, vomiting, fatigue, vertigo and weight loss (López-Pousa et al, 2007).

It is common practice to gradually withdraw the drug if the patient finds the side effects intolerable. The evidence regarding withdrawal is mainly from donepezil. Studies show that cognitive decline and appearance of adverse behaviours may occur following withdrawal, as the drug may still be having some clinical effect (Holmes et al, 2004). Therefore, a full clinical evaluation should be conducted when considering stopping or switching treatment, and it is important that all aspects of care are weighed and that the patient is reviewed at different points in time before the decision is made. If a trial of gradual withdrawal is considered then patients, carers and primary care health professionals are advised of the possibility of acute cognitive and behavioural deterioration, and the potential need to reintroduce medication promptly if worsening of symptoms is observed. It is important that patients are regularly reviewed by specialist services to provide holistic advice on management and care, particularly as Alzheimer's disease is a progressive condition. This is reinforced by NICE, which recommend regular follow up for these patients (NICE, 2011).

Polypharmacy in the older person

Major considerations in the care of the older person include comorbidity and polypharmacy. It is vital to assess and monitor kidney and liver function in this patient group as physiological changes due to age increase the risk of drug interactions and toxicity. The most commonly used drugs – acetaminophen, ibuprofen and aspirin – are available over-the-counter and contribute significantly to adverse drug reactions in the elderly. Generally, the more drugs a person takes, the greater the risk of adverse reactions and drug interactions. The drug categories most commonly involved in adverse drug interactions are cardiovascular agents, antibiotics, diuretics, anticoagulants, hypoglycaemic drugs, steroids, opioids, anticholinergics, benzodiazepines and NSAIDs. There are few main drug interactions with cholinesterase inhibitors. Research evidence suggests that medications with anticholinergic properties (such as some antipsychotics, antidepressants, anti-arrhythmia and antihistamine drugs) can affect the efficacy of cholinesterase inhibitors. Concomitant use of anticholinergic medication is seen in about 35 per cent of patients (Carnahan et al, 2004; Herrmann et al, 2007). Patients with Alzheimer's disease deserve to receive the optimum benefit from cholinesterase inhibitor treatment, which can only be achieved through diligent and appropriate use of concurrent pharmacotherapy.

Antipsychotic therapy in the care of the older person

There is little evidence of efficacy for use of antipsychotic drugs in the care of the older person to treat neuropsychiatric and behavioural symptoms (such as apathy, aberrant motor behaviour, appetite disturbance, irritability, agitation, wandering, aggression, sleep disturbance, depression, anxiety, delusions, disinhibition, hallucinations), which can manifest in patients with Alzheimer's disease. Risperidone is the only neuroleptic licensed for short-term use in patients with agitation and a review of the patient should take place after five to six weeks on treatment. Antipsychotics are widely used for many of the other symptoms listed but evidence for efficacy is lacking and there is the possibility that the antipsychotics may cause deterioration in cognitive function and increase morbidity and mortality in the older person. For example, older patients with dementia are particularly vulnerable to extrapyramidal and cardiac side effects of antipsychotic drugs. In the DART-AD trial (Ballard et al, 2009) maintenance on antipsychotics compared with termination of antipsychotic medication was associated with increased mortality. The study found that prolonged treatment resulted in up to 167 additional deaths among 1,000 people with dementia treated with antipsychotics over a two-year period. These findings suggest that mortality may increase with length of time taking antipsychotics for the older patient. Thus, antipsychotic drug use in the care of the older person should only be considered after carefully weighing the benefits and risks of treatment and should be for short-term use wherever possible. Generally, lower doses are recommended for older adults and, given the risk of drug interactions due to polypharmacy in this group, prescribers should always exercise vigilance. For people who are taking antipsychotic medication, weight, lipid profile, prolactin levels (if clinically indicated) and glucose levels, full blood profile (FBC, U&Es, LFTs) and presence of extrapyramidal side effects should be monitored and regularly assessed.

4.5 MEMANTINE (NMDA RECEPTOR ANTAGONIST)

Mechanism of action of memantine

Glutamate is another major excitatory neurotransmitter which acts on N-methyl-D-aspartate (NMDA) receptors found on membranes of nerve cells. Glutamate takes part in typical metabolic functions like energy production and ammonia detoxification as well as protein synthesis. Other functions include enabling neural communication, memory formation, learning and thinking. Increased levels of glutamate (overstimulation) leads to neural death, and it has been proposed that this could contribute to the cognitive symptoms present in Alzheimer's disease. Memantine is a NMDA receptor antagonist which irreversibly binds with the NMDA glutamate receptor and so selectively blocks glutamate transmission, thereby protecting neurons from excessive stimulation and death. It has been suggested that unlike other anti-dementia drugs, memantine does not have affinity for acetylcholinesterase enzyme, but instead exerts its neuroprotective effect on cholinergic neurons by blocking and downregulating the NMDA receptor activity.

In some studies, memantine was shown to improve the memory and behaviour of people with dementia in the medium and later stages of the disease (Winblad et al, 1999; McShane et al, 2006; Peskind et al, 2006). Memantine can be used for patients who are intolerant to cholinesterase inhibitors. Memantine's 5-HT3 antagonism may protect against the gastrointestinal side effects of cholinesterase inhibitors when used in combination therapy (Rammes et al, 2001).

Concomitant use of cholinesterase inhibitors and memantine

In a prospective study conducted at the University of Pittsburgh, 943 patients with Alzheimer's disease were evaluated and followed long term. The study compared patients receiving both memantine and cholinesterase inhibitors with patients receiving just cholinesterase inhibitors and patients receiving neither. The study found that patients treated with cholinesterase inhibitors had a decreased risk of institutionalisation compared with patients receiving no drug; and the patients who were treated with both memantine and cholinesterase inhibitors had the greatest decreased risk. The study findings show moderate benefits of combining cholinesterase inhibitors and memantine, including improvement in cognitions and functioning. The findings also showed that the combination therapy helped patients to stay longer in their homes and delay time to institutionalisation (Lopez et al, 2009). Gauthier and Molinuevo (2013) also report in their study that the combinations of memantine and donepezil produced significant benefits in cognition function, behavior, and care dependency, compared with donepezil treatment alone. NICE guidance (2018c) also recommends the use of memantine in combination with cholinesterase inhibitor in patients with an established diagnosis of Alzheimer's disease and in cases of moderate to severe Alzheimer's disease. The patient and their family or carers should be offered support and advice when combination therapy is considered. Clinicians with specialist skills and knowledge from either primary or secondary sectors should be consulted in involved in the planning and delivery of care.

Adverse effects and management of memantine

The most common adverse drug effects in patients taking memantine are dizziness, fatigue, headache, constipation, anxiety, somnolence, hallucinations and hypertension. Routine monitoring of side effects must include timely review of the patient, response to treatment and awareness of when polypharmacy may present increased risk of drug interactions. Withdrawal of medication should be tapered gradually, and the patient as well as carers must be informed of potential reoccurrence of symptoms following cessation of the medication.

The following screening and monitoring checks must be performed in the older patient taking anti-dementia drugs:

- FBC;
- urea, electrolytes and creatinine level;
- c-reactive protein (CRP);
- LFTs;
- TFTs;
- vitamin B12 and folate levels;
- vitamin D, calcium and bone profile;
- food and fluid monitoring;
- BMI and weight measures;
- memory testing;
- screening for depression, lifestyle factors (smoking, alcohol);
- blood pressure, pulse, temperature measures.

Case study 4 – Medication management

Background

Margaret is an 85-year-old woman with a diagnosis of Alzheimer's disease. Margaret currently lives with her husband but has recently been readmitted back to the inpatient older age ward following concerns that she has become withdrawn, has low mood and a reduced appetite. Margaret is currently taking donepezil as well as metformin for type 2 diabetes. Donepezil was started two months ago following Margaret's diagnosis. Margaret did not attend a review appointment with her GP before coming to the hospital and therefore missing having any health checks done. Her husband has reported that Margaret has been experiencing new symptoms of diarrhoea, dizziness, fatigue and hallucinations.

Care planning in the older adult with complex needs

Comorbidities such as anxiety, psychosis, physical health issues and depression in Alzheimer's disease are common. In this case study Margaret may be presenting with symptoms of a depressive illness (low mood, reduced appetite, withdrawn). The treating team will have to conduct a detailed assessment to rule out the presence of a depressive pathology in planning Margaret's care. Symptoms of depression in older people with dementia of any type could be triggered by the dementia; often the complexities and challenges of living with such health conditions may impact on the person's mental health and their well-being. Similarly, screening for more severe symptoms of mental illness is recommended especially when psychosis and its derivatives are suspected in this patient group. We can see that Margaret's husband is concerned about a new symptom – hallucinations – this would need to be considered by the treating team to screen Margaret for any presence of other psychotic symptoms. It is recommended to always assess the origin of such symptoms prior to starting pharmacotherapy. Not doing so may result in premature clinical decisions, ie co-administration of antipsychotics agents in older patients. In this case study, the new symptoms reported by Margaret's husband are likely side effects which are common in patients taking donepezil. In preparation for the review care planning meeting for Margaret, the team should consider the following interventions:

- *Assess the intensity and severity of side effects, and if the patient cannot tolerate these rivastigmine can be tried instead of donepezil. Rivastigmine is not known to cause neuropsychiatric reactions; however, side effects must still be discussed with the patient and their carer.*
- *Screening for depression would provide further information about Margaret's psychological well-being, and whether antidepressants may be considered in the management of depression if clinically indicated.*
- *Assess sleep hygiene and promote activities of daily living.*
- *Dementia review to assess disease progress and status.*
- *Offer carer's assessment for Margaret's husband.*
- *A full physical health screening must include:*
  - *FBC;*
  - *urea, electrolytes and creatinine level;*
  - *CRP;*
  - *LFTs;*
  - *TFTs;*
  - *vitamin B12 and folate levels;*
  - *vitamin D, calcium and bone profile;*
  - *food and fluid checks;*
  - *weight measures (including BMI);*
  - *screening for lifestyle factors (smoking, alcohol);*
  - *blood pressure, pulse, temperature measures;*
  - *blood glucose check and diabetic review.*

CHAPTER SUMMARY

Key points

- Anti-dementia drugs, also known as cognitive enhancers, are routinely used for the management of patients with Alzheimer's disease (the most common type of dementia) and other types of dementia.
- Biochemical abnormalities of acetylcholine and glutamate neurotransmitter systems in the basal forebrain (cerebral cortex and hippocampus) have been implicated in the aetiology and pathology of Alzheimer's disease.
- Pharmacological interventions for Alzheimer's disease include two drug classes including: acetylcholinesterase inhibitors (donepezil, rivastigmine, galantamine) and NMDA receptor antagonist (memantine).
- The older patient must be screened and offered interventions for common conditions that are known to cause cognitive, emotional and behaviour changes in this patient group including dehydration, infections, malnutrition, electrolyte derangements, anaemia, psychiatric illness, hypothyroidism, depression and any sensory impairment.

- Alzheimer's disease is a progressive and often irreversible disease which currently has no known cure.
- The common side effects associated with cholinesterase inhibitors and memantine include fatigue, dizziness, nausea, diarrhoea and vomiting.
- Polypharmacy is common in the care of the older patient; this carries a potential of various risks including adverse drug reactions and drug interactions. Clinicians must exercise vigilance to monitor and provide screening for unwanted drug effects, as well as being mindful to only prescribe further medication in situations in which the benefits clearly outweigh the risks posed to the patient.

CHAPTER 4 REVIEW QUESTIONS

Now have a go at answering these questions. You might find it useful to refer to the content of the chapter to locate the correct information for each question.

1. What symptoms are commonly associated with dementia?

2. Anti-dementia drugs are also known as _____. Fill in the missing words.

3. Antipsychotics and benzodiazepines can be adjunct treatment options to manage which symptoms of dementia?

4. Name two classes of drugs used to manage symptoms related to dementia.

5. What is the mechanism of action of acetylcholinesterase inhibitors?

6. What is the mechanism of action of memantine?

7. What is polypharmacy and of what relevance is this to an older patient?

8. Give examples of acetylcholinesterase inhibitors.

9. Describe the side effects associated with memantine.

10. Describe side effects associated with cholinesterase inhibitors.

11. What is acetylcholine?

12. What is glutamate?

13. Outline routine physical health checks/tests that should be conducted in older patients.

14. Name four drug groups commonly involved in drug interactions.

15. What anti-dementia drug is available in the form of patches?

16. What anti-dementia drug is available in the form of orodispersible tablets?

17. Generally speaking, the_____drugs a patient takes, the_____of adverse reactions and drug interactions. Fill in the missing words.

18. Memantine is licensed for treatment and management of _____Alzheimer's disease. Fill in the missing words.

19. Cholinesterase inhibitors often cure the symptoms of Alzheimer's disease. True or false?

20. What drugs does NICE recommend for the management of mild to moderate symptoms of Alzheimer's disease?

21. What risks are associated with the use of antipsychotics in patients with dementia?

22. Give three examples of drug classes that may interact with cholinesterase inhibitors.

23. Is there evidence that cholinesterase inhibitors can stop or reverse the process of nerve cell loss that causes Alzheimer's disease?

24. What is the indication for use of antidepressants in patients with Alzheimer's disease?

25. Name three different types of dementia.

Drugs used in bipolar disorders

5.1 INTRODUCTION

Bipolar disorder is a common and incapacitating mental disorder. This is a recurrent disorder which is characterised by repeated episodes of mania, hypomania or depression with complete inter-episode recovery. Mania is characterised by elated mood, overactivity, pressure of speech and disturbed sleep. Patients may show an increased speed of thought with enhanced productivity until efficiency or functioning is affected by poor concetration. Patients may experience hallucinations, mood-congruent delusions and irritability may occur rather the pure elation. Social inhibition, as well as social disinhibition, and unrealistic, extravagant and grandiose ideas – all of which may have negative consequences for the individual's life – have been reported. Depressive symptoms may include low mood, loss of interest, lethargy, poor concentration, apathy, social withdrawal, lack of apetitte, low self-esteem and confidence and are often accompanied by feelings of guilt, hopelessness and worthlessness. One-third of patients have chronic symptoms, and psychosocial difficulties are common.

Bipolar disorder has a global overall lifetime prevalence rate of 2.4 per cent (de Abreu et al, 2009; Merikangas et al, 2011). Bipolar disorder is a worldwide cause of disability and is ranked sixth in the world (Soreca et al, 2009). Bipolar I (type 1) disorder is considered the typical form of bipolar disorder, in which the patient experiences recurrent episodes of mania and depression. A wider, less well-characterised bipolar spectrum also exists which includes bipolar II (type 2) disorder in which the patient experiences a milder form of mania called hypomania (not frank mania) that alternates with depressive episodes, and cyclothymic disorder in which there is alteration in mood between hypomania and mild depression (not reaching severity of major depressive disorder). People with 'other specified bipolar and related disorders' also called 'subthreshold bipolar disorders', experience some elements of manic and depressive symptoms; however, the symptoms may not meet the strict criteria for any specific type of bipolar disorder noted in the Diagnostic and Statistical Manual of Mental Disorders, 5th edition (DSM-V; Severus and Bauer, 2013). Nevertheless, 'other specified bipolar and related disorders' can similarly lead to significant impairment (social, occupational and global) for patients.

Part of the criteria for efficacy and objectives of maintenance treatment is the prevention of new hypomanic/manic/depressive episodes, the optimisation of social and occupational functioning and minimisation of inter-episode symptoms (Taylor et al, 2012; Severus and Bauer, 2013). Mood stabilisers, benzodiazepines, anticonvulsant drugs, atypical and typical antipsychotics may be used to treat and manage acute mania, hypomanic and depressive symptoms. Antipsychotics such as risperidone, olanzapine, quetiapine, aripiprazole, asenapine are now commonly used as prophylactic first-line options for treatment of mania and hypomania (NICE, 2018a). This is due to the tranquillising and antimanic properties of these atypical drugs. However, the effectiveness of antipsychotics, as discussed in Chapter 2, is limited by their adverse metabolic effects (weight gain, blood dyscrasias, dyslipidaemia, cardiovascular and glucose abnormalities). Using a prophylactic antimanic agent augmented with an antidepressant is often a feasible option for long-term treatment in patients with bipolar disorder (Pacchiarotti et al, 2013). Benzodiazepines can also be used in acute manic emergencies to calm the agitated and highly elated patient. In addition, drug options in the management of acute episodes and for maintenance include lithium (which has the strongest evidence base of efficacy against mania), semisodium valproate or an atypical antipsychotic, for example olanzapine. However, lithium remains the drug of choice for many patients. It is recommended that the use of lithium, or anticonvulants such as valproate (sodium valproate and semi-sodium valproate), lamotrigine and carbamazepine, should only be initiated by a specialist psychiatrist in bipolar disorder in secondary care services; although primary care doctors may initiate such intervention with the guidance and support of a specialist and/or when there are shared care partnerships between primary and secondary care. General practitioners and others working in primary care are encouraged to refer patients they are concerned about to primary care mental health liaison teams (depending on local service delivery). Primary care mental health liaison teams have psychiatrists and specialist mental health nurses who can offer patient assessments within general practice premises.

Most, if not all, of the medications used to treat and manage patients with bipolar disorder have potentially severe adverse effects, and pharmacological choices may vary as the patient's symptoms and nature of their condition changes.

•   Medication choices will be different for female patients with bipolar disorder who become pregnant while on treatment. For example, lithium, valproate and carbamazepine drugs are all associated with an increased risk of foetal abnormalities (teratogenesis). Lithium treatment during pregnancy is associated with increased risk of congenital cardiac abnormalities in the foetus; and breastfeeding while on treatment is not recommended as lithium is found in breast milk. The use of carbamazepine or valproate anticonvulsants in the first trimester of pregnancy is associated with neural tube defects (abnormal opening/defects of brain, spine or spinal cord, ie spina bifida, anencephaly). Valproate is also reported to cause congenital digit and facial anomalies.

• As a minimum, effective contraception is essential for all women of childbearing age who are taking these medicines (Taylor et al, 2012). Moreover, NICE (2018a) recommends that valproate should not be regularly used to manage bipolar disorder in women of childbearing age, and that the prescriber should only consider using sodium valproate if nothing else works for the patient or if there are no safer alternatives. The risks and benefits of ongoing treatment should be carefully weighed, and the withdrawal of treatment should be undertaken prior to conception (MHRA, 2014). Therefore, pregnancy planning should be carefully co-ordinated in consultation with the prescribing psychiatrist to minimise potential risk to the developing foetus. In addition, special prenatal monitoring should be put in place, with the requirement to closely review the dose in pregnancy and after birth. However, more recently, NICE (2018a) has issued even stronger warnings about the teratogenicity of valproate, stating that this drug is associated with the highest risk and should not be used in women of childbearing age.

The primary choice of pharmacological intervention is based on whether the patient is manic or depressed, the severity of their symptoms, patient preference and the balance of benefit versus risk of adverse medication effects. The psychiatrist responsible for the patient's care is in charge of making treatment and management decisions regarding pharmacological approaches; he or she may prescribe additional medicines (benzodiazepines, antipsychotics) if required, eg when there is evidence in the patient's presentation of rapid cycling (presence of four or more distinct episodes of depression, mania, or hypomania occuring in one year), mixed states and/or psychotic symptomatology. The GP, carers, mental health nurses and other members of the MDT who may be involved in the care of the patient should alert the psychiatrist or the patient's clinical team of any changes in the patient's mood that might require a change in treatment. The care plan should be person-centred and aim to involve the patient, their family and carers.

In particular, patients and their carers should be educated in detecting early signs of manic episodes, eg increased activity or a decreased need to sleep, as well as the side effects of mood stabilising drugs (Culpepper, 2010). This is because patients who are manic may not feel they need treatment, and it is important to provide the patients and others involved in their care with continued advice and support around the benefits of taking medication, ensuring that their safety and that of others is prioritised with opportunities for regular reviews. Reducing stimulants, such as coffee, and avoiding the misuse of psychoactive substances (alcohol, cannabis, heroin) is advised, and it should be reiterated to patients that re-establishment of a healthy sleep regime is an important aspect of treatment (Malhi et al, 2010). NICE (2018a) recommends that patients with bipolar disorder presenting with depression in primary care should be offered a psychological intervention such as CBT, and there is evidence that in patients with bipolar I disorder medication plus cognitive therapy is more effective than medication alone for reducing relapses (Lam et al, 2005). Lithium, valproate and other mood stabilisers should only be initiated in primary care if there are clear developed shared care working partnerships between primary care and the secondary care mental health care services.

5.2 MECHANISM OF ACTION

Biochemical theories relating to the mechanisms within the brain by which symptoms of mania and depression manifest point to abnormalities in the neurotransmitter systems of noradrenaline, serotonin, dopamine and GABA. The monoamine hypothesis proposes that depressive features are associated with depleted/low levels of noradrenaline, and serotonin, while manic symptoms result from an excess of noradrenaline, serotonin, and low GABA neurotransmitters. This hypothesis is partly supported by findings of low levels of 3-methoxy-4-hydroxyphenylglycol (metabolite of noradrenaline) in the urine of depressed patients and low levels of serotonin metabolites found when post-mortems have been conducted in patients who have committed suicide. However, the mechanisms by which the neurochemical and neuronal changes induced by antidepressants and antimanic drugs are translated into clinically meaningful effects in bipolar and unipolar patients are still broadly unknown (Bhui et al, 1998; Catherine et al, 2009).

The mechanism of action underlying the mood stabilising effects of valproate, carbamazepine, lamotrigine and lithium is not clearly understood. It is postulated that carbamazepine may enhance serotonin transmission, but it is not clear whether sodium valproate or lamotrigine share the same mechanism. The anti-epileptic effects of valproate, carbamazepine and lamotrigine are thought to be the result of blockade of voltage-gated sodium channels, leading to reduction in neuronal membrane excitability. It is also suggested that valproate may enhance inhibitory GABA neurotransmission. A combination of these and other actions in the brain could explain the mood stabilising effects of these medications.

Lithium, valproate, carbamazepine and lamotrigine are regarded as the most venerable pharmacological options in the treatment and management of bipolar disorder. These medication options, particularly lithium, are regarded as first-line or newer atypical antipsychotics in cases where the patient has a new diagnosis of bipolar affective disorder. Valproate, lamotrigine and carbamazepine are anticonvulsants used in the management of epilepsy but also have mood stabilising uses.

NICE (2018a) guidelines recommend asenapine, haloperidol, olanzapine, quetiapine or risperidone as first line in the treatment and management of mania and hypomania. Asenapine is an atypical antipsychotic which is currently licensed only for the treatment of bipolar disorder.

5.3 DOSE AND ADMINISTRATION

Table 5.1 Examples of drugs used in bipolar disorder

Drugs	Type of drug	Indication	Oral dose range divided in two daily doses (mg)
Lithium carbonate (Camcolit, Liskonum, Phasal, Priadel)	Mood stabiliser	Mania Bipolar disorder Recurrent depression Aggressive or self-harming behaviour	200–1500 mg (Dose must be individualised and adjusted according to body weight and serum-lithium concentration)
Lithium Citrate Li-Liquid®	Mood stabiliser	Mania Bipolar disorder Recurrent depression Aggressive or self-harming behaviour	509–1018 mg for adults with body weights up to 50 kg 1018–3054 mg for adults with body weights 50 kg and above 509–1018 mg for the elderly (Dose must be individualised and adjusted according to body weight and serum-lithium concentration)
Lithium Citrate Priadel® liquid	Mood stabiliser	Mania Bipolar disorder Recurrent depression Aggressive or self-harming behaviour	510–1040 mg for adults with body weights up to 50 kg 1040–3120 mg for adults with body weights 50 kg and above 510–1040 mg for the elderly (Dose must be individualised and adjusted according to body weight and serum-lithium concentration)
Sodium Valproate (Depakote)	Anticonvulsant	Mania	750–2000 mg

(continued)

Table 5.1 (*Cont.*)

Drugs	Type of drug	Indication	Oral dose range divided in two daily doses (mg)
Carbamazepine (Tegretol, Carbagen)	Anticonvulsant	Prophylaxis of bipolar disorder unresponsive to lithium	400–1600 mg
Lamotrigine	Anticonvulsant	Monotherapy or adjunctive therapy of bipolar disorder	100–400 mg (100–200 mg adjuctive with valproate and max 400 mg without valproate)

Lithium

Lithium salts such as lithium carbonate, lithium citrate and lithium orotate are mood stabilisers. Lithium has been used for over 60 years for the treatment of bipolar disorder (recurrent mania/hypomania and depression) and is still frequently prescribed. Unlike most other prophylactic antimanic drugs, lithium can counteract both mania and depression. Lithium can also be used to augment other antidepressant drugs in patients with treatment-resistant depression (in patients whose depressive symptoms have shown partial or no response to anti-depressants). Lithium is licensed in the UK for the treatment of aggressive or self-harming behaviour. Occasionally, lithium is prescribed as a preventive treatment for migraine disease and cluster headaches. The active principle in these salts is the lithium ion, which by having a smaller diameter, can easily displace potassium and sodium and even calcium ions, occupying their sites in several critical neuronal enzymes and neurotransmitter receptors. The mood stabilising effect has been hypothesised to relate to a decrease in catecholamine neurotransmitter concentration, perhaps mediated by lithium ion influence on the important membrane pump sodium/potassium adenosine triphosphatase (Na^+/K^+-ATPase), to create improved trans-neuronal membrane transport of sodium ions (Quiroz et al, 2010). Equally, it has been established that lithium possesses several effects on central neurotransmission, most importantly in relation to the modulation of presynaptic monoamine neurotransmission or interaction with intracellular second messenger systems as well as neurotransmitter receptors (Malhi et al, 2009). Other theories have been proposed for the mood stabilising effects of lithium; however, the exact mechanism underlying the therapeutic efficacy of lithium in bipolar disorder remains unclear (Malhi et al, 2013).

Lithium is indicated for the treatment of mania, hypomania, prophylaxis of bipolar disorder and recurrent depression. Lithium can also be used to treat aggression and suicidality. The full prophylactic and therapeutic effect of lithium may be delayed by up to four to seven days following initiation of therapy; hence an antipsychotic such as olanzapine may be used in the acute phase of mania or hypomania for patients who experience frequent relapses and continued functional impairment. However, the co-administration of antipsychotics can increase the risk of neurological side effects (Taylor et al, 2012). The clinical team should offer regular assessments and reviews and enquire about potential neurological and metabolic side effects that may be associated with combination therapies. Lithium is more effective at preventing mania than depressive relapse (Geddes et al, 2004). NICE (2018a) recommends lithium as a first-line combination therapy for patients who have been offered and tried an antipsychotic (asenapine, haloperidol, olanzapine, risperidone and quetiapine) in secondary care for the management of mania and hypomania.

Dose and administration of lithium

The usefulness of lithium is limited by its adverse effects, narrow therapeutic window and patients' non-adherence to treatment. All patients taking lithium will require ongoing laboratory blood and physical health checks and monitoring; prescribers and other health care professionals involved in the care of patients taking lithium will need to consider potential drug interactions and adverse side effects that may arise. The long-term use of lithium has been associated with thyroid complaints, as well as moderate cognitive and memory impairment. Therefore, long-term treatment should be considered only with careful monitoring and weighing up of risks and benefits for the individual patient.

Lithium is usually started at 300–400 mg at night (200 mg in the elderly), and subsequently the dose is adjusted to maintain plasma blood lithium levels within the desired range of 0.4–1.0 mmol/L. Plasma lithium level should be taken after seven days, then seven days after every dose change, and taken until the desired level is reached (0.4 mmol/L may be effective in unipolar depression, 0.6–1.0 mmol/L in bipolar disorder, slightly higher levels in difficult-to-treat mania; Taylor et al, 2012). Blood samples should be taken 12 hours after the last dose. For patients in secondary and primary care, it is common for the lithium blood test to be taken usually in the early hours of the morning after the previously given evening dose and before administering the morning dose.

Lithium is available in two forms: lithium carbonate (tablets) and lithium citrate (liquid). Importantly, the lithium carbonate tablet and the lithium citrate liquid are not equivalent, so doses cannot be applied interchangeably between preparations. Therefore, when prescribing and administering, lithium needs to be prescribed by brand due to wide differences in bioavailability. Even within each preparatory form of lithium, marked variation exists, and the changes in how an individual will metabolise the different brand of drug cannot be reliably predicted. Therefore, care must be taken when prescribing and administering lithium, such that the patient receives their usual brand of drug; but also, prescribers must view any change in preparation as a dose change, and so the same monitoring of blood lithium levels and precautions should apply.

Upon initiation of lithium, patients will be provided with a lithium treatment pack to continuously record and monitor the patient progress on lithium. The pack can be used to record blood test results (lithium levels) and other blood measures. Also included is a lithium alert card that is to be kept by the patient at all times to show they are on a lithium treatment regime.

Valproate

Also known as valproic acid, this anticonvulsant drug is used in both psychiatric and non-psychiatric conditions. In the UK, valproate is available in three preparations: valproic acid, sodium valproate and semi-sodium valproate (Taylor et al, 2015). The former is approved for the management of epilepsy, while the latter two preparations are licensed for the treatment of acute mania; both semi-sodium and sodium valproate are metabolised to valproic acid, which plays a role in the pharmacological action of all three preparations (Fisher et al, 2003). According to a large open maintenance trial of patients with rapid cycling, sodium valproate was effective both as monotherapy but also when used in combination with lithium (Calabrese et al, 1990). This drug is effective in patients with acute mania and may even be better than lithium in patients with dysphoric mood (Andres et al, 1999). These findings indicate efficacy and generally good tolerability of sodium valproate in maintenance treatment, with effectiveness at least comparable to lithium. NICE (2018a) recommends valproate as a second-line combination intervention with an antipsychotic if lithium does is ineffective. Valproate plasma level monitoring is allegedly less useful than with lithium or carbamazepine therapy; however, plasma levels can be used to detect non-adherence or to monitor toxicity in patients.

Dose and administration of valproate

The usual daily dose ranges from 750–2000 mg, in one to two divided doses; lower doses are recommended in the older patient. Treatment is usually started at low doses and increased steadily at three-day intervals until the desired level is reached. The commonly reported side effects are reduced when the doses are gradually titrated. Valproate has a relatively short drug half-life (eight to 12 hours); hence the drug may need to be taken two to three times a day to maintain a steady blood concentration. Sodium valproate has been associated with liver injury and thrombocytopenia at high doses; as such, LFTs and FBCs, including platelet levels, should be tested every six to 12 months to reduce the risk of toxicity. Blood tests should be conducted immediately before the first daily dose. Any patients with raised LFTs (common in early treatment) should be assessed clinically and other indicators of hepatic function such as albumin and clotting time should be checked (Bjornsson, 2008). Sodium valproate should be used with caution in patients with pre-existing liver disease. Unlike lithium, sodium valproate can be used for long-term maintenance therapy with fewer side effects.

Carbamazepine

Carbamazepine is an anticonvulsant yet it is structurally like TCAs. It is widely used to treat and manage partial seizures, generalised tonic-clonic seizures, pain of neurological origin, such as trigeminal neuralgia, and as a prophylactic agent in the treatment and management of bipolar disorder in patients who may be unresponsive to other mood stabilising drugs. In the UK it is licensed for the treatment of bipolar disorder in patients who do not respond to lithium. NICE (2018a) recommend that carbamazepine should be used in patients unresponsive to a combination of other prophylactic antimanic drugs, ie antipsychotics combined with lithium. Carbamazepine is generally considered to be more useful in patients who experience more than four affective episodes (mania, depressive episodes or hypomania) a year. A common term used to refer to this is rapid cycling.

The mode of action of carbamazepine is not fully understood, although it is proposed that the drug inhibits sustained repetitive firing of neurons, by blocking use-dependent sodium channels and therefore reduces glutamate release (a key excitatory neurotransmitter in the brain). Therefore, carbamazepine possesses muscle relaxant, sedative and antidepressant properties (possibly also through antagonism of noradrenaline release), as well as anticholinergic, central antidiuretic and anti-arrhythmic effects. It has similar efficacy potential to lithium in the treatment of acute mania, but it can take up to 14 days to produce a significant clinical response. Carbamazepine may be useful as a prophylactic agent for the treatment of bipolar disorder in patients in the following instances:

* rapid cycling disorder (four or more affective episodes in a year);
* unipolar depression either alone or as an augmentation strategy (Zhang et al, 2008);
* patients who have poorly responded to lithium therapy;
* mania with mixed states (anxiety and depression);
* patients with comorbid epilepsy;
* schizoaffective disorder;
* patients who cannot tolerate the side effects of other mood stabilisers.

Dose and administration of carbamazepine

Carbamazepine is usually started at 400 mg daily in one to two divided doses, with the dose gradually increased as required until symptoms are controlled (usually 400–600 mg daily), up to a maximum of 1600 mg daily. A lower dose is recommended in older patients, in patients with multiple physical comorbidities and in patients with smaller body size/lower body weight. The titration should be done over a period of one to two weeks to lessen the incidence and severity of side effects such as nausea, dizziness and vomiting. It is important to note that the modified-release formulations can be given once to twice daily, and these slow-release tablets are associated with reduced fluctuations in serum levels and are generally better tolerated by patients. Carbamazepine has a drug half-life of 16–24 hours and as such the dose is usually split into twice-daily dosing.

Carbamazepine has been associated with agranulocytosis, a serious and potentially life-threatening condition resulting from a deficiency of granulocytes (a class of white blood cells), causing elevated vulnerability to infection. FBCs and LFTs should be done before treatment and at least three to six weeks after starting treatment, and thereafter when there are clinical symptoms such as fever, ulcers or infection. It is also good practice to use plasma levels monitoring to ensure adequate dosing and treatment compliance. Most importantly, the dose range should be checked in the first month of commencing treatment because carbamazepine is a potent inducer of hepatic cytochrome P450 enzymes (alters the rate of drug metabolism in the liver), and therefore results in subsequent increase in the metabolism of carbamazepine itself after four weeks' administration. This leads to a consequential reduction in the blood levels of carbamazepine even when the patient's dose has not changed. Hence, the prescriber may need to consider increasing to a higher dose, but it is important to note that the required dose increase will be individually specific and so will vary between patients. (Please refer to Chapter 2, and the section titled 'Prescribing antipsychotic drugs to smokers' [subheading under Section 2.3 'Dose and administration'], for further details about enzyme inducers and hepatic cytochrome P450 metabolism.) In patients with bipolar disorder, a dose of at least 400 mg per day and a plasma level of at least 4 mg/L is the target, with levels above 12 mg/L significantly associated with higher side effects (Taylor and Duncan, 1997). If carbamazepine is to be discontinued, it should be done slowly.

NICE (2018a) recommend that U&Es, FBCs and LFTs should be repeated after six months, and that weight (or BMI) should also be monitored in patients on carbamazepine therapy. The responsibility of monitoring should be a multidisciplinary approach; nurses, doctors and other mental health professionals must equally share this responsibility and highlight to others in the team any areas in relation to best practice found to be sub-standard.

Lamotrigine

Lamotrigine is an anticonvulsant drug, licensed in the UK for the treatment of both epilepsy and bipolar disorder. Like other mood stabilisers, the mode of action of lamotrigine is poorly understood, but it is suggested that lamotrigine works by blocking sodium channels on nerve cells. Lamotrigine can be used as a monotherapy for bipolar disorder or in conjunction with other mood stabilising drugs (eg valproate, lithium or carbamazepine). There is evidence that lamotrigine is particularly effective in the treatment and management of bipolar depression and that it can treat depressive presentations in patients without causing mania, rapid cycling or hypomania.

Dose and administration of lamotrigine

Therapeutic dosing of lamotrigine needs to be up titrated slowly. As monotherapy, lamotrigine is initiated at a dose of 25 mg daily for 14 days; then increased to 50 mg daily in one to two divided doses for a further 14 days; then the dose is increased to 100 mg daily in one to two divided doses for a further seven days; and thereafter mainte-nance dose is typically 200 mg daily in one to two divided doses (maximum of 400 mg daily). Lamotrigine has relatively few side effects and does not require blood monitor-ing. However, reports of lamotrigine-induced insomnia are common, so if the patient is on a once-a-day dosing schedule then it is recommended to take the medication in the morning. Caution is advised when prescribers are adding or removing other drugs to a patient's treatment regimen, as dose adjustments for lamotrigine may be subsequently required.

5.4 ADVERSE EFFECTS, MONITORING AND MANAGEMENT

Lithium

Adverse effects, monitoring and management

Lithium has a narrow therapeutic index (little difference between therapeutic and toxic doses) and therefore should not be given to patients unless there are services available for monitoring lithium serum levels. Patients should have FBCs, U&Es, serum creatinine, estimated glomerular filtration rate (eGFR), LFTs, TFTs, calcium levels, urinalysis, base-line BMI and ECG conducted pre-treatment.

For assessment of serum lithium levels while on treatment, blood samples should be taken 12 hours post-dose administration; with the target range being 0.4–1.0 mmol/L (lower end of range for older patients and for maintenance therapy). Patients need to be informed that on the morning of their lithium blood test, they should not take lithium until the blood sample has been collected. A slightly higher target serum–lithium dose range of 0.8–1.0 mmol/L is recommended for acute episodes of mania and for patients that have previously relapsed (BNF, 2018c). However, it is good practice to determine the optimum range for each patient by regular clinical review of psychiatric symptoms as well as any reports of side effects. For the prophylaxis of bipolar disorder, most prescribers prefer a serum range of about 0.6–0.8 mmol/L; some patients may require higher doses, but these doses are associated with higher risk of adverse effects. Blood levels should be measured weekly for the first eight weeks or until the levels stabilise, and every two to three months during maintenance. Patients should also be told that if they forget to take a dose; they should never take a double dose to make up for the missed dose but wait and take their usual prescribed dose at the next due time.

It is good practice to check U&Es, eGFR, creatinine calcium levels, TFTs, ECG and monitor weight/BMI every three to six months. Additional serum lithium levels should be tested if the patient develops a significant change in sodium and/or fluid intake, as hyponatraemia and/or dehydration can induce lithium toxicity. More frequent testing may also be required in patients who are prescribed interacting drugs. When lithium is being withdrawn, dosing should be reduced gradually over a month and it is good practice to do follow-up blood tests for lithium levels upon stopping lithium treatment.

Adverse effects

- Metallic taste in the mouth.
- Nausea and diarrhoea – common in first few weeks and then usually settles. If these symptoms reappear or persist when treatment is established, this may indicate toxicity.
- Weight gain.
- Lithium can cause a reduction in urinary concentrating capacity – nephrogenic diabetes insipidus; hence patients report symptoms of polyuria (increased urination) and polydipsia (increased thirst and drinking excessive fluids).
- Some skin conditions such as psoriasis and acne can be aggravated by lithium therapy.
- Tremor – if problematic, can be treated with co-administration of propranolol (beta blocker) tablets.
- Ankle oedema.
- Lithium increases the risk of hypothyroidism; in middle-aged women, the risk may be up to 20 per cent (Johnston and Eagles, 1999). If it occurs, hypothyroidism is easily treated with levothyroxine tablets or by stopping lithium.
- Long-term treatment with lithium can lead to cognitive and memory impairment.
- Lithium is associated with increased risk of cardiac foetal abnormalities, particularly if treatment is continued during the first trimester of pregnancy. Lithium also has the potential to cause harmful, toxic effects on breastfeeding infants and so should be avoided in lactating mothers.

PRECAUTIONS

Due to lithium's relatively narrow therapeutic window, pharmacokinetic interactions with other drugs can often lead to lithium toxicity (Juurlink et al, 2004; Stockley, 2018). Of note, the most significant interactions are with drugs that alter renal sodium handling, such as NSAIDs, thiazide diuretics, and angiotensin-converting enzyme (ACE) inhibitors. Additionally, prescribers need to exercise caution in the co-administration of lithium and SSRIs, as a common side effect of the latter is hyponatraemia, which can then precipitate lithium toxicity. Prior to starting or stopping any medication, patients should be encouraged to always seek expert advice from their doctor or pharmacist, and declare all medications, including those not prescribed, such as over-the-counter medicines, any herbal preparations and drugs bought online. It is a professional responsibility of all mental health professionals to enquire about medication history and allergies in the planning of every patient's care.

Lithium toxicity

Lithium salts have a narrow therapeutic index, with serum lithium concentration levels greater than 1.5 mmol/L most likely to lead to toxic effects, and levels greater than 2.0 mmol/L associated with serious toxicity and may be life-threatening. Mild toxicity can be reversed by the administration of copious amounts of sodium and fluids; more severe toxicity may require haemodialysis.

Initial symptoms of mild to moderate lithium toxicity are usually:

- gastrointestinal symptoms, such as:
  - increasing anorexia;
  - vomiting;
  - nausea;
  - polyuria;
  - diarrhoea;

and

- CNS symptoms, such as:
  - muscle weakness;
  - drowsiness;
  - ataxia (lack of co-ordination);
  - coarse tremors;
  - dysarthria;
  - muscle twitching.

Dangerous lithium concentration levels greater than 2 mmol/L leads to:

- acute renal failure;
- increased risk of disorientation and confusion;
- cardiac arrhythmias;
- convulsions (seizures), which can progress to coma, and ultimately death.

It is important to educate the patient about early warning signs of toxicity and to not ignore symptoms reported by the patient, eg vomiting, drowsiness, diarrhoea and polydipsia. The most common cause of toxicity is dehydration, which is usually caused by hot weather leading to loss of fluid through sweating or when the patient is physically exhausted. Other causes include: reduced dietary intake of sodium, urinary tract infections, kidney disease, accidental overdose and co-administration of drugs which inhibit the rate of lithium excretion from the body or alter renal sodium handling (diuretics, NSAIDS, ACE-inhibitors). Lithium therapy should not be withdrawn suddenly as evidence suggests this may increase the likelihood of relapse. Rather, withdraw lithium slowly over several weeks and reassess regularly for relapse.

Case study 5 – Management of lithium toxicity

Background

Steve is a 25-year-old male with a diagnosis of bipolar disorder. He is a current inpatient on a general psychiatric ward but has daily leave to the community grounds. On admission to the ward Steve was taking lithium 800 mg daily. The ward consultant reviewed Steve's medication during the last MDT meeting and the daily dose of lithium was increased to 1000 mg. This is Steve's ninth day on the new dose. Today, Steve returns from his community leave and complains to the nurse that he has been feeling sick while walking in the park near the hospital grounds. Steve reports to the nurse that he has vomited twice, has ongoing nausea and has increasing muscle pain and weakness. Steve appears more drowsy than usual and his care record shows a significant increase in the frequency of trips Steve has been making to the toilet over the past few days.

Care planning for lithium toxicity

Lithium is very effective in the treatment and management of mania in bipolar disorder, but its use is limited in practice due to lithium's narrow therapeutic window and the drug's toxic effects on the body. In this case study, the nurse caring for Steve will have to be well informed about the adverse effects of lithium toxicity in order to spot the early warning signs. As discussed above, in the sub-chapter on lithium, the symptoms reported by Steve are typical of lithium toxicity (nausea, vomiting, drowsiness, muscle weakness, polyuria/diarrhoea) and if Steve does not receive the right support and interventions to address this, toxicity may lead to seizures, coma with hyperreflexia (a condition in which the body's involuntary nervous system overreacts to external or bodily stimuli) and even death. The MDT must consider the following points in Steve's care plan to effectively manage lithium toxicity in this case:

- *The clinical team must stop further administration of lithium and assess Steve for any other signs of toxicity, eg ataxia, nystagmus, dysarthria, tremors and epileptic seizures.*
- *A blood test to check serum lithium levels in Steve's body should be conducted and assessed at least every six hours; we know that the toxic syndrome occurs at levels above 1.5 mmol/L.*

- *Other blood tests including urea and electrolytes, serum creatinine, FBC, TFTs and LFTs should be conducted.*
- *An ECG should be performed to check cardiac rhythm and function.*
- *Steve will require adequate fluid and sodium intake. The nurse should strongly encourage Steve to drink plenty of fluids, and he will likely require supplementation with intravenous fluids also. Furthermore, Steve's sodium levels need to be maintained within the normal range; aim for sodium levels of 140–145 mmol/L.*
- *Urine output must be measured, and a fluid balance chart maintained.*
- *The nurse should encourage the patient to remain on the ward until his condition stabilises and it is deemed safe to re-establish community leave.*
- *To minimise risk of falls or other harm to Steve, the nurse should allocate another member of staff to stay with Steve and continuously monitor him; any signs of further deterioration should be escalated to a senior member of staff and the medical team should be urgently alerted.*

Valproate

Adverse effects, monitoring and management

Common side effects, particularly with starting doses above 750 mg daily include:

- nausea and vomiting;
- diarrhoea;
- sedation;
- headache.

Less common side effects include:

- hair loss/alopecia;
- weight gain – can be especially problematic if valproate is used in conjunction with atypical antipsychotics such as olanzapine or clozapine;
- ankle oedema;
- pancreatitis;
- thrombocytopenia;
- hepatic failure;
- ataxia;
- tremor.

Some of these symptoms may be reversible when valproate is discontinued.

PRECAUTIONS

- Valproate can increase serum warfarin concentrations and facilitate bleeding by interfering directly with platelet function and coagulation processes (Stephen, 2003).
- Hepatic failure resulting in fatalities has occurred in patients receiving valproate and its derivatives. These incidents usually occur during the first six months of treatment. Serious or fatal hepatotoxicity may be preceded by non-specific symptoms such as malaise, weakness, lethargy, facial oedema, anorexia and vomiting. In patients with epilepsy, a loss of seizure control may also occur. Patients should be monitored closely for appearance of these symptoms. Serum liver tests should be performed prior to therapy and at frequent intervals thereafter, especially during the first six months.
- Sodium valproate should not be prescribed to patients who have liver failure/dysfunction.
- Valproate is contraindicated in pregnancy as it can cause major congenital malformations, particularly neural tube defects (eg spina bifida), but also facial malformations (eg cleft lip and palate) and malformations of the limbs, heart and kidney. Additionally, in utero exposure to valproate has been associated with children having decreased IQ scores and increased risk of autism spectrum disorders.
- Valproate should not be administered to women of childbearing age due to the high risk of serious developmental disorders (up to 30–40 per cent risk) and congenital malformations (approximately 11 per cent risk; BNF, 2018d; MHRA, 2018). The MHRA in the UK has published a safety valproate toolkit for guidance purposes for all organisations providing NHS and private health care to alert clinicians and all female patients of childbearing potential of the serious teratogenic risk valproate possesses to the unborn child.
- If there are no other safe alternative options, female patients must use effective contraception while using valproate. Prescribers seeking to use valproate in female patients of childbearing age will have to ensure that the conditions of the 'Pregnancy Prevention Programme' are met, as set out by MHRA (2018), before the medication is used. This includes the completion of risk acknowledgement form, signed by both the patient and a specialist, and reviewed at least annually.
- Cases of life-threatening pancreatitis have been reported in both children and adults taking valproate. Some of the cases have been described as haemorrhagic with rapid progression from initial symptoms to death. Some cases have occurred shortly after initial use; others after several years of use. Patients and carers should be warned that abdominal pain, nausea, vomiting and/or anorexia can be symptoms of pancreatitis, and require prompt medical evaluation. If pancreatitis is diagnosed, valproate should be discontinued.

- Valproate should not be used in conjunction with aspirin or carbamazepine because of harmful drug interactions. Other known interactions are with psychotropic drugs including phenothiazine and clonazepam. It is important to take a drug history from the patient before prescribing; this must be included in both doctor and nurse assessment.
- Sodium valproate may enhance the effects of CNS depressants such as alcohol, barbiturates, general anaesthesia and other anticonvulsants, ie pregabalin.

Carbamazepine

Adverse effects, monitoring and management

The side effects below are common with carbamazepine use, and are usually present at the commencement of treatment, though they tend to subside after a few days. They can sometimes be minimised by starting with a low dose and titrating slowly. High peak blood levels of carbamazepine can be avoided by splitting the dose throughout the day or by using a modified-release formulation.

Common side effects:

- nausea and vomiting;
- hyponatraemia (abnormally low sodium levels in the blood);
- dry mouth;
- oedema;
- sedation (dose-related; may improve with dose reduction);
- constipation or diarrhoea;
- CNS toxicity – dizziness, ataxia, visual symptoms, headaches (these are usually dose related);
- skin rashes or hives – these may indicate an allergic reaction usually evident after one to two weeks following commencement of treatment. The drug should be stopped.

A less common, but serious adverse effect of carbamazepine is a low white blood cell (leukopenia) or neutrophil count (neutropenia), with one patient in 20,000 developing potentially life-threatening agranulocytosis and/or aplastic anaemia (Joan et al, 2006). Patients should be educated and asked to urgently report any of following symptoms:

- paleness of skin;
- bleeding;
- mouth ulcers;
- weakness;
- fever;

- any signs of infection;
- sore throat;
- cough;
- bruising easily;
- vomiting;
- abdominal pain or inflammation of the liver (hepatitis).

Please refer to Chapter 2, and the section titled 'Haematological adverse effects' (subheading under Section 2.4 'Non-extrapyramidal adverse effects of antipsychotic drugs') for further details about drug-induced blood disorders.

PRECAUTIONS

- The metabolism of other drugs (including carbamazepine itself) may be accelerated because carbamazepine is a cytochrome P450 enzyme inducer. Of importance is the enhanced metabolism of hormonal contraception (eg combined oral contraceptive pill), which leads to a reduction in contraceptive efficacy. Female patients taking carbamazepine and requiring contraception should either receive a preparation containing at least 50 µg of oestrogen and twice the amount of progestogen (and take the oral contraceptive pill every day, without the usual seven-day break each month), or use a non-hormonal method of contraception.
- Plasma levels of most antidepressants, most antipsychotics, benzodiazepines, some cholinesterase inhibitors, methadone, thyroxine, theophylline and steroids may be reduced by carbamazepine (due to its enzyme-inducing action), resulting in treatment failure.
- Drug agents that inhibit CYP3A4 enzyme will increase carbamazepine plasma levels and may precipitate toxicity, for example cimetidine, diltiazem, verapamil, erythromycin and some SSRIs. Nurses and doctors are advised to make a full enquiry of all the medicines prescribed to their patient, as well as those obtained over-the-counter or bought online to fully assess for potential drug interactions.
- Carbamazepine is contraindicated in patients with cardiac atrioventricular (AV) conduction abnormalities and porphyria.
- Carbamazepine is a known human teratogen; an agent that can disrupt the normal development of an embryo or foetus. There is an increased risk of congenital foetal malformations, especially spina bifida, if carbamazepine is taken during pregnancy.
- In female patients of childbearing age, if carbamazepine cannot be avoided through the use of an alternative safe medication, effective contraception should be observed (note the interaction between carbamazepine and oral contraceptives as discussed above) and prophylactic folate co-prescribed (BNF, 2014).

- The likelihood of carbamazepine to cause neutropenia may be increased by concomitant use of other drugs that also have the potential to depress the function of the bone marrow (eg clozapine, doxorubicin, methyldopa-hydrochlorothiazide).
- The risk of hyponatraemia may be increased by other drugs that have the potential to deplete sodium levels in the blood (eg diuretics, SSRIs).
- Though rare, neurotoxicity has been reported when carbamazepine and lithium are used concurrently.
- Before starting and during treatment with carbamazepine, the following tests should be conducted as best practice: FBCs, U&Es, LFTs, ECG and weight/ BMI.

Lamotrigine

Adverse effects, monitoring and management

The common side effects associated with lamotrigine include:

- dizziness;
- headaches;
- insomnia;
- lack of co-ordination;
- blurred vision;
- nausea;
- vomiting;
- body aches and cramps;
- drowsiness;
- dry mouth;
- changes in appetite;
- skin rashes and fever in the first weeks of treatment.

Very rarely, lamotrigine has been known to cause a severe skin reaction called Stevens-Johnson syndrome (SJS), which tends to occur more often in children and adolescents than adults, when lamotrigine is used as anti-epileptic drug. This condition is also likely to occur during dose increases; so, it is recommended to titrate lamotrigine slowly over a few weeks during treatment to avoid causing the reaction. SJS usually begins with flu-like symptoms and fever, followed by painful and blistering rash of the skin and mucosal surfaces of eyes, mouth and throat. Mental health nurses caring for patients starting this drug or patients already taking this drug should exercise awareness and screen patients accordingly. Similarly, the occurrence of any rash reported by the patient or observed by the nurse early in treatment should lead to further assessment and evaluation, and consideration of stopping the treatment. Compared to other antimanic drugs (mood stabilisers), lamotrigine is among the safer drugs for use during pregnancy; a study of 3000 mothers taking it in pregnancy showed that the drug does not significantly increase the risk of birth defects during pregnancy (Wise, 2017).

PRECAUTIONS

- Toxicity is likely when valproate is used alongside lamotrigine, as the combination leads to an increase in lamotrigine levels.
- Carbamazepine, due to its enzyme-inducing action, has been known to lower lamotrigine levels.
- Women are more likely than men to experience side effects of lamotrigine; this might be due to interaction between lamotrigine and the female hormones. Also, lamotrigine may become less effective due to changes in the body during pregnancy; hence the patient's dose may need to be increased by approximately 25 per cent compared to the pre-pregnancy dose.
- In lactating mothers, lamotrigine is present in breast milk, but usually only in small amounts, and not generally considered to be at sufficient levels to affect the baby (Dalili et al, 2015).
- Drug-induced blood disorders (aplastic anaemia, bone-marrow failure) have rarely been associated with lamotrigine.
- Patients should be encouraged to report any signs and symptoms of hypersensitivity reactions; although in some cases hypersensitivities might occur without a rash or skin reaction. Other signs may include: fever, puffiness of the face and swollen lymph glands.
- Patients with bipolar disorder taking lamotrigine should be advised against stopping the drug suddenly, to reduce the risk of relapse of depressive episode.

CHAPTER SUMMARY

Key points

- Bipolar disorder is a recurrent disorder which is characterised by repeated episodes of mania, hypomania or depression with complete inter-episode recovery.
- Biochemical theories implicate abnormalities in neurotransmitter systems of the brain including serotonin, noradrenaline, dopamine and GABA in the pathology of bipolar disorder.

- Antimanic, also known as mood stabilising drugs (lithium, carbamazepine, valproate, lamotrigine), as well as antipsychotic drugs, antidepressants and benzodiazepines are used in the treatment and management of bipolar disorder.
- The incidence of metabolic adverse effects increases in combination therapies, therefore close monitoring of the patient, particularly serum drug levels in patients taking lithium and/or carbamazepine, is essential to minimise risk and harm to patients taking these psychotropic agents.
- Lithium has a narrow therapeutic range; serum lithium concentrations above the range associated with toxicity requires urgent identification and management.
- Due to risk of teratogenicity, both lithium and valproate should be avoided in female patients of childbearing age; if there are no alternative treatments, prescribers must be cautious and ensure effective contraception in female patients of childbearing age is a key point to remember.
- Carbamazepine has been associated with agranulocytosis, a potentially serious and life-threatening reaction to the drug which requires prompt assessment, treatment and management.
- Physical health checks should be conducted, including measures, pulse and blood pressure, blood glucose, glycosylated haemoglobin (HbA1c) and blood lipid profile, liver function, renal profile and TFTs.

CHAPTER 5 REVIEW QUESTIONS

Now have a go at answering these questions. You might find it useful to refer to the content of the chapter to locate the correct information for each question.

1. Name the common symptoms reported by patients with mania.

2. Is breastfeeding recommended in women on lithium therapy for bipolar disorder?

3. What checks should be conducted before initiating lithium therapy?

4. Why is monitoring serum lithium concentration important in patients?

5. Can you give examples of symptoms associated with lithium toxicity?

6. State the target serum lithium concentration range, within which lithium is at safe and effective levels.

7. What mood stabiliser does NICE recommend as first-line management of acute mania and bipolar disorder for patients in secondary care?

8. Antipsychotics are routinely used solely or in combination with mood stabilisers in the treatment and management of bipolar disorder. True or false?

9. What risks are associated with the use of antidepressants in bipolar disorder?

10. What is a teratogen?

11. Carbamazepine and clozapine are both known to cause agranulocytosis. What does this term mean?

12. Give examples of three antipsychotic drugs that may be used in the management of bipolar disorder.

13. What does the abbreviation 'FBC' stand for in full and what does this test measure?

14. Does lithium have a narrow or a wide therapeutic index? What does this mean for you as a health professional?

15. What are some symptoms of mild to moderate lithium toxicity?

16. Name a mood stabiliser which is a potent cytochrome P450 enzyme inducer.

17. Why is it important for doctors and nurses to always ask about a patient's past and current medication history?

18. Teratogenicity means that lithium and carbamazepine should be avoided in___ _____. Fill in the missing word.

19. What are the common side effects associated with the use of carbamazepine and sodium valproate?

20. Can sodium valproate be prescribed to patients with liver dysfunction?

21. What worrying symptoms may be present in a patient on carbamazepine with a low WBC count?

22. What medical condition(s) is valproic acid indicated for?

23. What is the usual daily dose range of sodium valproate?

24. Psychotic symptoms are common in patients with bipolar disorder. True or false?

25. Why should prescribers avoid withdrawing lithium suddenly in patients with bipolar disorder?

Drugs used in anxiety disorders

CHAPTER AIMS

This chapter covers:

*   the symptomatology of anxiety;
*   the role of GABA neurotransmitter in the aetiology of anxiety;
*   the mechanism of action of anti-anxiety drugs;
*   different groups and types of anti-anxiety drugs used in mental health settings;
*   the adverse effects associated with anti-anxiety drugs;
*   recommended monitoring and management of drug adverse effects.

6.1 INTRODUCTION

Benzodiazepines sometimes called 'benzos' are a class of drugs that are often used clinically as sedatives, anxiolytics, hypnotics, anti-epileptics or muscle relaxants depending on the metabolism profile of the drug preferred and the dose used. It is common to find benzodiazepines prescribed alone or in combination with other medications used to treat mental health disorders, such as antidepressants, anti-dementia drugs, antipsychotics and mood stabilisers. However, recently, NICE (2018a) found no evidence to support the use of benzodiazepines alongside antidepressants in the initial treatment of depression. Also, NICE (2011) recommends that benzodiazepines should not routinely be used in patients with panic disorder, as in comparison the benefits from CBT or SSRIs, used alone or in combination, are far superior.

Anxiety is usually co-morbid with other pathologies including depression, eating disorders, psychoses or substance abuse. First-line interventions are usually psychotherapeutic interventions involving cognitive therapies, counselling, relaxation techniques, mindfulness cognitive-based therapies and self-help strategies. Patients with typical anxiety disorders such as generalised anxiety disorder (GAD), panic disorder and/or social anxiety disorder often report the following symptoms:

*   feeling weak, faint or dizzy;
*   racing heart (palpitations);
*   chest pains;

- breathing difficulties;
- tingling or numbness in the hands and fingers;
- feeling sweaty or having chills;
- feeling of loss of control;
- sense of terror or feeling of impending doom or death.

Anti-anxiety drugs (also known as anxiolytics) are commonly used to treat moderate to severe symptoms of anxiety but will also induce sleep when administered at bedtime; hypnotics are indicated for the treatment of insomnia and will produce sedative effects if administered during the day. Hypnotic drugs usually have shorter half-lives compared to the longer half-life of anxiolytics. The half-life of a drug is how long it takes for half of the dose of the drug to be eliminated from the bloodstream. Short half-life drugs (eg lorazepam) are more likely to result in rebound insomnia and anxiety when the drug is stopped, and they may also cause temporary memory difficulties. Long half-life drugs (eg diazepam) require less frequent dosing and have more stable plasma blood concentrations, and so they tend to be associated with mild withdrawal symptoms compared to short half-life drugs. However, it is important to note that long half-life benzodiazepines can cause increased daytime drowsiness and can lead to greater plasma concentrations of the drug in the body and result in a higher risk of psychomotor impairment. Other differences between benzodiazepines are the length of time it takes a drug to produce the desired effects (onset of action), and the amount of the drug needed to achieve a specific effect (potency).

Sedative drugs produce a calming effect for the agitated or anxious patient while anxiolytics may reduce the excessive levels of anxiety. Hypnotics cause drowsiness and may be used to induce sleep. In the UK, apart from benzodiazepines, hypnotic drugs are not licensed for the treatment of anxiety. Importantly, the use of both benzodiazepines and hypnotics in the management of anxiety and insomnia is limited by the high risk of these drugs to cause tolerability and dependence (both physical and psychological). Withdrawal effects can occur upon stopping the drug, especially after prolonged administration. Hence, it is recommended that both benzodiazepines and hypnotics should only be used for short-term treatment regimens (not to be prescribed for longer than one month) to manage acute presentations after specific precipitating or causal factors have been identified. The use of benzodiazepines should be avoided in those patients with a history of major personality difficulties and patients with a history of substance misuse.

Older anxiolytics such as barbiturates are not recommended; tolerance to barbiturates occurs more rapidly compared to benzodiazepines, physical dependency may occur even at very small doses and these drugs have far more side effects and drug interactions than benzodiazepines. Furthermore, barbiturates are more dangerous in overdose; for these reasons, benzodiazepines have replaced barbiturates as hypnotics and sedatives of choice (Scott and McGrath, 2009).

Benzodiazepines are commonly administered orally but may be administered parenterally (intravenous or intramuscular injection) in some clinical situations, for example when a highly agitated/distressed patient possesses a risk of causing harm to themselves or others and needs rapid sedation. Like most drugs, benzodiazepines are metabolised in the liver and primarily excreted via the kidneys in the urine. The liver plays a major role in metabolism, digestion, detoxification and elimination of substances from the body. Enzymes in the liver are responsible for chemically changing drug components into substances known as metabolites. The clinical team should ensure that before administration of benzos or other psychiatric drugs a physical health examination is undertaken; blood tests, LFT, hepatic function, FBC, thyroid function tests and assessment for medical conditions known to cause anxiety symptoms should be investigated and properly addressed.

6.2 MECHANISM OF ACTION

Benzodiazepine hypnotics and anxiolytics

Benzodiazepines target and stimulate the benzodiazepine receptors (benzodiazepine binding site) on gamma-aminobutyric acid-A (GABA$_A$) receptors, located on the membranes of postsynaptic neurons at many sites within the CNS, including the limbic system and ascending reticular activating system (RAS) of the brain. The RAS is linked to wakefulness and attention; GABA is the main inhibitory neurotransmitter in the brain, it is the brain's most abundant inhibitory, or 'calming', neurotransmitter and plays a role in regulating many aspects of mood, attention, cognition and sleep. GABA deficiency symptoms have been associated with depression, anxiety, insomnia and others. The interaction between benzodiazepines and GABA receptor site is complex, but ultimately leads to the potentiation of GABAergic transmission and dampening of neuronal excitability due to increased membrane permeability to chloride ions. This shift in chloride ions results in hyperpolarization of the neuron, which is a less excitable state and inhibits action potentials. Consequently, the resulting increase in inhibitory transmission is thought to denote the whole spectrum of the therapeutic actions of benzodiazepines.

As mentioned earlier in this chapter, benzodiazepines are metabolised in the liver and some are broken down into one or more active metabolites; this action effectively prolongs their duration of action. They are classified into short-acting (three to eight hours), intermediate-acting (six to 20 hours) and long-acting (one to three days) drugs, depending on the relative durations of action. Hypnotic drugs with a rapid onset of action (time to effect) and shorter duration of action are usually preferred in the treatment of insomnia, while longer-acting drugs are preferred in the treatment and management of anxiety.

Non-benzodiazepine hypnotics

'Z-drugs', which include zopiclone, zolpidem, zaleplon and eszopiclone, are benzodiazepine receptor agonists. These drugs work in a similar way to the benzodiazepine drugs inside the brain at the GABAergic receptor sites, but they are chemically different in structure to benzodiazepines. As these drugs act as GABA agonists, they increase the inhibitory neurotransmission of GABA, and thereby induce sleepiness. Some evidence suggests that they only interact with a subset of GABA receptors, which may explain their enhanced selective hypnotic effect (Rudolph and Mohler, 2014). Historically in the treatment of insomnia, the Z-drugs were developed after the benzodiazepines.

Barbiturates, like benzodiazepines, increase GABAergic transmission by their action on GABA receptor sites. They target and bind to the barbiturate binding site on the receptor, an action which increases neuronal inhibitory GABAergic transmission activity. Nowadays, barbiturates (such as phenobarbital and sodium thiopental) are no longer routinely used in the treatment of insomnia or anxiety as discussed above; however, they are still sometimes used for general anaesthesia in surgery and in the treatment of epilepsy.

Antihistamine sedatives, such as promethazine, are antagonists at H1 receptors in the CNS, with consequences including drowsiness and sedative effects. Promethazine also has antiemetic, anticholinergic and weak antipsychotic properties, which are clinically beneficial, for example reducing symptoms of nausea and psychosis, but also contribute to a wide range of side effects, including headaches, dry mouth, constipation, blurred vision and psychomotor deficits. The prolonged duration of action of drugs such as promethazine and chloral hydrate can often result in daytime drowsiness the following day post-administration. The precise mode of action of chloral derivatives (eg chloral hydrate) in inducing sleep remains unclear.

Melatonin

Melatonin in the UK is only licensed for use in adults over 55 years of age. Melatonin is a hormone made by the pineal gland situated in the middle of the brain. Melatonin is involved in helping the body to recognise sleep and waking; the body naturally produces this hormone but supplements containing melatonin are now commonly used. With age, the amount of naturally occurring melatonin reduces and so consuming pharmacological or herbal supplements of the hormone can increase the body's natural capacity and helps to promote and improve sleep.

Non-benzodiazepine anxiolytics

Non-benzodiazepine anxiolytics include buspirone and beta blockers, antidepressants, antipsychotics and anticonvulsants. Buspirone is less sedating than other anxiolytics and is thought to be a partial agonist at specific serotonin (5-HT1A) receptors. At this location, 5-HT1A receptors function as inhibitory auto-receptors regulating serotonin neuronal activity. It is the 5-HT1A agonist properties of buspirone that may explain its anxiolytic action. Buspirone has a slow onset of action and patient response to buspirone can be delayed by up to two weeks. However, unlike benzodiazepines, its use does not usually lead to drug dependence, nor does it lead to withdrawal effects upon stopping. Additionally, it is less sedative and does not cause usually CNS depressant effects when combined with alcohol or other CNS depressant drugs. Patients who are used to the sedative effects of benzos may not find buspirone useful as it lacks sedative effects.

Table 6.1 Comparison of benzodiazepine and buspirone

Benzodiazepine	Buspirone
Rapid onset of action	Delayed onset (not appropri-
Can induce sedation	ate for PRN use)
Can cause dependence and withdrawal	Does not induce sedation
Pharmacokinetic change with age	Non-addictive
May impair performance	No pharmacokinetic change with age
Drug interaction with CNS depressants	Does not impair performance
Significant additive CNS depres-	No drug interaction with
sant effects with alcohol	CNS depressants
Associated with falls in the elderly	Minimal additive CNS depres-
	sant effects with alcohol
	Not associated with falls in the elderly

Evidence of efficacy backs the use of some atypical anticonvulsants in the treatment and management of anxiety, ie gabapentin, vigabatrin and pregabalin (Mutsatsa, 2015). Specifically, pregabalin has been studied and found to be effective in the treatment and management of GAD. Pregabalin structurally inhibits the breakdown of GABA neurotransmitter, thereby increasing GABAergic inhibitory neurotransmission in the brain. Pregabalin also modulates the release of many excitatory neurotransmitters such as glutamate and noradrenaline. This modulation can cause an inhibitory regulation of overexcited neurons enabling them to return to a normal state. This neurotransmitter regulation could explain pregabalin's anxiolytic as well as its anticonvulsant activity (Rajappa et al, 2016).

Many of the antidepressant medications are also licensed for use in a wide range of anxiety disorders including GAD, panic disorder, OCD, post-traumatic stress disorder (PTSD), social anxiety disorder and agoraphobia (see Chapter 3, Table 3.1). In particular, SSRIs (such as sertraline, escitalopram, paroxetine), TCAs (such as nortriptyline, amitriptyline), as well as mirtazapine, venlafaxine and trazodone, are examples of antidepressant medications that are often used to good effect in patients with anxiety. Please refer to Chapter 3 for more details about these antidepressants.

Beta blockers, such as propranolol and oxprenolol, act as antagonists at betaadrenoceptors located in the sympathetic nervous system. They are clinically useful in managing somatic symptoms related to anxiety and panic disorder (eg palpitations, tremor, sweating) but do not have any clinical effect on the psychological symptoms of anxiety. These drugs are sometimes used in conjunction with SSRIs for the treatment and management of depression and neurotic-related conditions.

Trifluoperazine is a typical antipsychotic drug that may be used to treat schizophrenia and psychosis but is also indicated for the management of severe anxiety at lower doses. Please refer to Chapter 2 for more details about typical antipsychotics.

6.3 DOSE AND ADMINISTRATION

Table 6.2 Examples of benzodiazepines and non-benzodiazepines used in the management of insomnia and anxiety

Class	Further class details	Examples of drugs	Oral dose range (mg/daily)
Benzodiazepines used in insomnia	Intermediate-acting	Temazepam	10–20 mg
	Intermediate-acting	Loprazolam	1–2 mg
	Long-acting	Nitrazepam	5–10 mg
	Long-acting	Flurazepam	15–30 mg
Benzodiazepines used in anxiety	Short-acting	Oxazepam	15–120 mg
	Intermediate-acting	Lorazepam	Anxiety:1–4 mg daily in divided doses. Insomnia: 1–2 mg before bed For rapid tranquillisation (RT), maximum is 4 mg in 24 hours. Oral and IM are the same dose but must be written separately on chart. Mix lorazepam with 1:1 water for injection before administering. For elderly halve the normal adult dose
	Long-acting	Diazepam (Valium)	2–30 mg
	Long-acting	Chlordiazepoxide (Librium)	15–100 mg
	Long-acting	Clobazam	20–60 mg
	Long-acting	Clonazepam	Panic disorder 1-2 mg

			Clonazepam IM (unlicensed in the UK) is an alternative for RT. Licensed in Canada and New Zealand. IM dose is like oral 500 mcg–2 mg Maximum 4 mg in 24 hours. Mix the clonazepam 1:1 with the water for injections before injecting. Administer a concentration of 500 mcg/ml
Non-benzodiazepines used in insomnia	Z-drugs	Zopiclone	3.75–7.5 mg
		Zolpidem	5–10 mg
		Zaleplon	5–10 mg
	Anti-histamine, neuroleptic	Promethazine	25–50 mg
	Hypnotic	Chloral hydrate	400–2000 mg
	Hypnotic, naturally-occurring hormone	Melatonin	2–5 mg
Non-benzodiazepines used in anxiety	Anxiolytic	Buspirone	10–45 mg
	Antidepressants	SSRIs TCAs Venlafaxine Trazodone	See Chapter 3, Table 3.1
	Atypical anticonvulsant	Pregabalin	150–600 mg
	Typical antipsychotic	Trifluoperazine (Stelazine)	2–6 mg
	Beta-blockers	Propranolol	40 mg once daily, increased if necessary to 40 mg three times a day.
		Oxprenolol	40–80 mg daily in one or two divided doses (short-term use).

6.4 ADVERSE EFFECTS AND MANAGEMENT

Adverse effects of benzodiazepines

The most important unwanted effect of benzodiazepine administration is related to risk of both psychological and physical dependence, potential for abuse and tolerance, as noted earlier in this chapter. In Australia, the survey by the National Drug Authority (AIHW, 2013) found that tranquillisers and sleeping pills, including benzodiazepines were the second most commonly misused medicine behind painkillers/analgesics. Diazepam and lorazepam are some of the most commonly abused benzos in the UK and the United States. To this end, benzodiazepine administration is recommended for use for short periods of time, generally between two to four weeks. Short-acting benzodiazepines are also associated with acute withdrawal symptoms such as increased anxiety, agitation and tremors; these often occur the morning following evening administration. When weaning patients off benzodiazepines following prolonged use, gradual dose tapering is always recommended. Short-acting benzos (eg lorazepam) may be associated with withdrawal effects that can last up to 7 days and for long-acting drugs (eg diazepam [valium]) withdrawal effects can last up to 90 days following long-term use.

Other side effects associated with benzodiazepines are:

- daytime sedation (with all benzodiazepine anxiolytics);
- 'morning hangover effect' (with all classes of hypnotics);
- amnesia;
- ataxia (poor co-ordination);
- impaired reaction time and impaired performance (can affect driving ability and ability to operating machinery);
- fatigue;
- dry mouth;
- nausea and vomiting;
- muscle weakness;
- dizziness;
- adverse mood effects (depression, emotional anaesthesia, aggression);

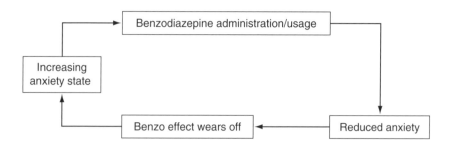

Figure 6.1 Dependency cycle of benzodiazepines

- disinhibition (seems more common with shorter-acting drugs);
- use in the elderly is associated with increased vulnerability to confusion, memory impairment, over-sedation and risk of falls;
- respiratory depression (less common and dose-related – also more likely with intravenous administration).

Paradoxical reaction

Occasionally benzodiazepines induce a paradoxical reaction marked by agitated delirium with emotional lability, hostility, aggression and restlessness. These effects may also include: over-excitement, increased rate of speech and anti-social acts (BNF, 2014). Risk factors for paradoxical reactions are prevalent in people with psychiatric comorbidity, learning disabilities, neurological disorders or CNS degenerative diseases, alcoholism and the elderly. The risk is further increased if the benzodiazepine is a high-potent drug, given in a high dose or when given intravenously (Bond, 1998).

Treatment consists of discontinuing the offending agent and flumazenil can be used if indicated to reverse the reaction. If needed, non-GABA drugs may be used (eg ketamine, haloperidol and opioids) if not contraindicated (Cabrera et al, 2010). Failure to recognise and treat paradoxical reactions might lead to a vicious cycle of ongoing agitation (Mancuso et al, 2004).

Withdrawal from benzodiazepines

When stopping benzodiazepines, it is important to consider the following:

- Sudden stopping of benzodiazepines is dangerous as it increases the risk of seizures; hence benzodiazepines should always be gradually tapered and not terminated abruptly.
- Withdrawal symptoms can occur between doses; it is common for patients to believe that these symptoms are related to their original anxiety problems.
- Symptoms of withdrawal can include increased anxiety, insomnia, aching limbs, nausea, nervousness, restlessness, irritability, fatigue, delirium, tremors and depression.
- Short half-life benzodiazepines are associated with more acute and intense withdrawal symptoms.
- Withdrawal symptoms for long half-life benzodiazepines tend to be mild and more delayed in onset.
- Symptoms of withdrawal can be experienced by patients discontinuing low-dose benzodiazepines as well as patients on high doses.
- There is generally a low risk of developing tolerance, dependence and withdrawal when drugs are used sparingly and in moderate doses for only one to two weeks.
- Mental health professionals must exercise vigilance to recognise signs of problematic drug use, such as drug-seeking behaviour and patterns of elevated or escalating use of drugs.

Managing withdrawal symptoms

- Ensure the dose of benzodiazepine is reduced slowly, with regular patient reviews to monitor for early symptoms of withdrawal, such that dosing can be adjusted as required.
- Implement relaxation, cognitive and breathing techniques.
- Refer to drug and alcohol services for patients with co-occurring drug and alcohol complex care needs.
- Refer to primary psychological services to access CBT or other psychological interventions where clinically appropriate.
- Offer the patient reassurance that the symptoms are usually temporary.
- If managed withdrawal is proving to be difficult for the patient, despite the low evidence base switching to diazepam is recommended for some patients, particularly they are taking short-acting drugs or having difficulties withdrawing (Taylor et al, 2012).
- The rate of benzodiazepine withdrawal should be determined for each patient, bearing in mind the drug, dose, duration of treatment, withdrawal symptoms and patient factors (eg personality, lifestyle, previous experiences and co-morbid medical/psychiatric and psychological problems).

Risk of overdose with benzodiazepines

- Benzodiazepine overdose can occur when a patient takes more than the recommended dose or if the patient combines the benzo drug with another central nervous depressant substance, such as alcohol, opioids, barbiturates or TCAs.
- Signs and symptoms of overdose include dizziness, confusion, drowsiness, blurred vision, hypotension, respiratory depression, altered mental status, bluish fingernails and lips, disorientation and coma.

Treatment in overdose

- Flumazenil is a selective benzodiazepine receptor antagonist. Flumazenil binds to the GABA receptor at the benzodiazepine binding site, but does not induce the action of GABA, ie it has no effect. In doing so flumazenil displaces any benzodiazepine present on the receptor, thus reversing the action of the benzodiazepine.
- Flumazenil has a short duration of action, so if the patient has taken a large overdose of benzodiazepines they may experience re-sedation and recurrent respiratory depression once the effects of flumazenil wear off. Hence, repeated administration may be required.
- As flumazenil is a benzodiazepine antagonist, its administration can precipitate withdrawal symptoms in the patient.
- It is important to note that flumazenil is dangerous to use if the patient has a mixed overdose (particularly benzodiazepines taken with TCAs, carbamazepine or amphetamines), as it can result in convulsions and cardiac arrhythmias. Patients who have taken an overdose are often poor at keeping records, so if you are not entirely confident of all the drugs taken, it is often safer to avoid using flumazenil.

- It is essential to closely monitor patients who have taken an overdose, including: pulse, blood pressure, respiratory rate, oxygen saturation, temperature, ECG, blood tests (FBCs, U&Es, creatinine, LFTs, clotting, lactate, blood gases, glucose level, and alcohol levels).
- Seeking urgent medical attention in a timely manner is important to reduce the potential of adverse consequences and death.

Adverse effects of non-benzodiazepine hypnotics

Z-drugs

Like benzodiazepines, evidence shows that zopiclone and zolpidem also induce dependence; therefore, it is recommended that Z-drugs are only used for short periods (usually up to four weeks).

Other common side effects of the Z-drugs are:

- gastrointestinal upset;
- dizziness;
- bitter taste (commonly reported in patients taking zopiclone);
- headaches;
- 'morning hangover effect' (with all classes of hypnotics);
- fatigue;
- dry mouth.

Management of the side effects may involve adjusting the patient's dose, changing the time of administration or changing to a shorter-acting drug to overcome some of these problems. It is also important for clinicians to take a comprehensive drug history from the patient including historic or current use/dependence on alcohol and other illicit substances. Assess for drug interactions and adverse reactions and always consider a non-pharmacological intervention first to manage the patient's anxiety or insomnia. CBT has been shown to improve sleep quality, reduce hypnotic drug use and improve health-related quality of life among long-term hypnotic users with chronic sleep difficulties (Jacobs et al, 2004). Mental health nurses should ask the patient about possible side effects associated with the use of hypnotics during one-to-one review meetings, as well as regular assessment to check whether the drug is still required. Generally, the assessment should check for any drug seeking behaviours or tendencies – for example, where the following are suspected:

- patients asking for early prescription renewal;
- patients seeking and aggressively requesting higher doses of hypnotics or benzodiazepines;
- when patients obtain similar drugs from different sources;
- selling prescription drugs;
- patients increasing doses without clinical advice;

- repeatedly losing prescriptions;
- buying drugs from the Internet to supplement their prescriptions;
- stealing or borrowing from friends/family.

Promethazine

Common adverse effects that have been reported in patients taking promethazine include:

- dizziness;
- tinnitus;
- ataxia;
- blurred vision;
- restlessness;
- dry mouth
- headache;
- skin rashes;
- urinary retention;
- constipation.

Rare but potentially serious side effects of promethazine include:

- arrhythmias;
- blood disorders;
- anaphylaxis;
- depression;
- hypotension;
- liver dysfunction;
- convulsions;
- extrapyramidal side effects.

Precautions and interactions (benzodiazepines and hypnotics)

- Most sedative and hypnotic drugs will interact with other CNS depressants (including alcohol and opioids) to produce an increased sedative effect.
- Benzodiazepines and hypnotics should not be used in patients with liver disease, a history of substance abuse, during pregnancy or in people performing hazardous tasks, eg operating machinery, driving or performing tasks that require mental alertness.
- The metabolism of some benzodiazepines is inhibited by the following drugs: erythromycin, oral contraceptives, zopiclone, diltiazem, anti-fungals, cisapride, cimetidine and verapamil. This may result in increased plasma concentrations of benzodiazepines and increased or prolonged sedation as well as increased side effects.
- Conversely, the metabolism of some benzodiazepines is induced by other drugs, including: rifampicin, St John's Wort (herbal antidepressant) and some anti-epileptic drugs (eg carbamazepine, phenytoin) resulting in decreased sedation.

- Benzodiazepines and hypnotics should be used sparingly in the elderly and monitored due to increased risk of adverse effects (cognitive deficits, falls, disinhibition, agitation).
- Patients should be advised of the risk of rebound insomnia when a hypnotic is stopped.
- Hypnotics should not be used in sleep apnoea.
- Advise patients to avoid driving or operating heavy machinery until it is established whether the medication makes them drowsy during the daytime or not.

Case study 6 – Medication management and unhealthy lifestyle behaviours

Background

Fred is a 30-year-old male with a diagnosis of major depression and panic disorder. He has a history of abusing alcohol when he is feeling depressed. He lives with his wife and three kids (8, 5 and 2 years of age). His wife reports that recently Fred has been experiencing poor sleep, reduced appetite and that he won't leave the house because of fear of experiencing panic attacks. Fred also becomes anxious around people and in crowded public places. He is currently on the maximum daily dose of citalopram as well as a daily dose of diazepam 10 mg. His wife has recently stopped giving Fred diazepam as he has started excessively drinking alcohol again. Fred lacks insight and does not recognise that he is becoming unwell. Without his wife's knowledge, Fred has gone to see his GP to request for another prescription of diazepam. However, he is unaware that his wife has already informed the GP about Fred's current relapse in mental health functioning which is further complicated by problematic abuse of alcohol.

Care planning in complex case presentations

Anxiety in depression and vice versa is common as both conditions are known to induce clinical features reported in both depressive and chronic anxiety pathologies. There may be tendencies in both pathologies to exhibit reckless behaviour and patients may be prone to abuse drugs and alcohol particularly, if there is a past history. Patients may not recognise they are depressed and so may fail to seek help; and if there is a history of addictive personality and maladaptive behaviours, then re-emergence of drug-seeking behaviours is almost inevitable. Of note, in Fred's case, a combination of diazepam and alcohol use should be avoided because both drugs enhance GABA levels in the brain and can result in increased sedation, drowsiness and CNS depression. Fred's historic and problematic use of alcohol coupled with current concerns expressed by his wife could explain why Fred has attended his GP to ask for more diazepam; both diazepam and alcohol are known to induce tolerance and therefore create dependence in users. Fred's wife was right to not administer diazepam and to inform his GP about the current relapse. By going to see his GP, Fred's doctor will have the opportunity to conduct a detailed clinical assessment of Fred's mental health and well-being and assess whether Fred uses other illicit substances such as cannabis, crack or heroin. An alcohol screening tool (eg Alcohol Use Disorders Identification Test, AUDIT-C) could be conducted to assess how much Fred drinks. Fred's doctor could ask about Fred's mood, thinking and understanding of current needs, psychosis, physical health status, as well as questions around self-harm and suicidal thoughts that are usually part of any mental state examination. The GP will likely undertake a further, more detailed assessment to ascertain whether Fred's anxiety may be related to dependence on diazepam or whether this is due to panic disorder. Also, the GP should discuss with Fred about medication adherence regarding citalopram and any other prescribed drugs, as well as providing education on health dangers resulting from harmful alcohol use, drug interaction with diazepam, and non-adherence to prescribed medication.

Fred's scenario provides some insight into managing typical complex cases in primary care; management of such cases requires a MDT approach and interprofessional working partnerships. For example, with Fred's consent, the GP may need to refer Fred to the drugs and alcohol team for further management and support, community psychology (once Fred's alcohol use is under control), and the secondary care mental health team could be consulted regarding a medication review. Moreover, a carer's assessment should be offered to Fred's wife, and it is important not to forget to ensure safety and welfare of the children, which is paramount.

Adverse effects of non-benzodiazepine anxiolytics

Buspirone

The common side effects of buspirone are:

* dizziness;
* excitement;
* headache;
* nausea;
* nervousness.

To avoid hypertensive reactions, buspirone should not be used in combination with MAOIs. Furthermore, buspirone can increase the risk of serotonin syndrome, and so caution is needed if co-prescribing with antidepressant drugs. Please refer to Chapter 3, and the sections titled 'Monoamine oxidase inhibitors' and 'Serotonin syndrome' (sub-headings under Section 3.4 'Adverse effects and management') for further details.

Buspirone is not recommended in patients with severe hepatic or renal impairment. It is licensed for short-term use only in the UK; however, it is not uncommon for specialist prescribers to use it for several months.

Pregabalin

The most common adverse effects reported from pregabalin use are:

* dizziness;
* somnolence;
* peripheral oedema;
* nausea;
* headaches;
* blurred vision;
* dry mouth;
* diarrhoea;
* increased appetite and weight gain.

Abrupt withdrawal of pregabalin should be avoided; reducing the dose should be tapered over at least one week if the drug is to be stopped.

Beta blockers (propranolol)

Reported side effects of beta blockers are:

* bradycardia;
* breathlessness;
* coldness of hands and/or feet;

* dizziness;
* headaches;
* hypotension;
* gastrointestinal disturbances.

Beta blockers are contraindicated in patients who have asthma or obstructive airways disease, due to the risk of bronchospasm. In addition, these drugs should be avoided in pregnancy as they can cause hypoglycaemia, bradycardia and growth restriction in the baby.

CHAPTER SUMMARY

Key points

* Anxiolytics are used for the treatment and management of severe anxiety, while hypnotic drugs are indicated for the short-term treatment of insomnia.
* Most anxiolytic drugs are thought to increase GABA inhibitory neurotransmission in the brain, a desired effect for the anxious or agitated patient.
* Drug treatment of both anxiety and insomnia is limited by the potential for anxiolytic drugs (eg benzodiazepines) and hypnotic drugs (eg zopiclone) to induce tolerance and dependence. It is always best to consider a non-pharmacological intervention first to manage the patient's anxiety or insomnia.
* Withdrawal from benzodiazepines can produce a state characterised by increased agitation, sweating, tremors and anxiety; abrupt cessation of benzodiazepines is dangerous as this can cause seizures. Benzodiazepines should always be gradually tapered to minimise or avoid withdrawal symptoms.
* Monitoring physical health is important to screen and address drug side effects and interactions, especially when there is combination therapy with other drugs such as antipsychotic drugs, mood stabilising agents or antidepressants.
* The speed of benzodiazepine withdrawal should be determined for each patient, bearing in mind the drug, dose, duration of treatment, withdrawal symptoms, and patient factors (eg personality, lifestyle, previous experiences and medical/psychiatric and psychological co-morbidities).

CHAPTER 6 REVIEW QUESTIONS

Now have a go at answering these questions. You might find it useful to refer to the content of the chapter to locate the correct information for each question.

1. What are some of the clinical uses of benzodiazepines?

2. It is common to find benzodiazepines co-administered with an antipsychotic drug. True or false?

3. What is drug half-life? What is drug potency?

4. Give an example of a benzodiazepine with a long half-life and one with a short/intermediate half-life.

5. Give examples of six different drugs from at least three different classes that are licensed for the treatment of anxiety in the UK.

6. What are the major clinical concerns and issues related to prolonged use of anxiolytics and hypnotics?

7. What are the clinical manifestations of a paradoxical reaction to benzodiazepines and which groups of people are mostly at risk?

8. Barbiturates are commonly used in clinical practice for the treatment of anxiety disorders in the UK. True or false? What is the rationale for your answer?

9. What are the symptoms of benzodiazepine withdrawal?

10. Benzodiazepines with_____half-lives are associated with more acute and intense withdrawal symptoms compared to benzodiazepines with_____ half-lives. Fill in the missing words.

11. In which organ of the body are drugs often converted into metabolites?

12. What is the main inhibitory neurotransmitter in the brain?

13. Give three examples of non-benzodiazepine hypnotics.

14. What is the name of the receptor site for Z-drugs?

15. Name the antihistamine drug that may be used in the management of insomnia. What are the common side effects associated with this drug?

16. List three differences between buspirone and benzodiazepines.

17. Give two examples of beta blockers. What are the clinical benefits of using beta blockers in patients with severe anxiety?

18. Name an antipsychotic drug that is also licensed for use in severe anxiety in the UK.

19. What is the usual daily dose range of diazepam and lorazepam?

20. What is the name of the drug that can be given (with caution) to reverse the effects of benzodiazepines?

Appendix

ANSWERS TO CHAPTER REVIEW QUESTIONS

Chapter 1

1. What are antipsychotic medications?
   ✓ Antipsychotic medications are pharmacotherapeutic agents used to manage and control the symptoms related to a diagnosed mental disorder such as schizophrenia, bipolar disorder, transient psychotic presentations and psychotic depression.

2. What other name is usually used to refer to antipsychotic drugs?
   ✓ Neuroleptics.

3. What is the stress–vulnerability model and how does it contribute to the understanding behind aetiology of mental illness?
   ✓ The model suggests that when stress factors and intrinsic biological/vulnerability factors interact beyond a threshold, mental illness emerges.

4. What is a neuron? Give another name for a neuron.
   ✓ A neuron is a functional unit of the central nervous system (CNS). Most commonly, neurons are also referred to as nerve cells.

5. Where do nerve impulses or chemical reactions originate from?
   ✓ Within the neuron.

6. What is the space between two neurons called?
   ✓ Synaptic cleft.

7. What do you call the cubicles where neurotransmitters are found?
   ✓ Synaptic vesicles.

8. What is the main difference between the presynaptic and postsynaptic neuron?
   ✓ The onset of a nerve impulse originates from the presynaptic neuron to excite the release of neurotransmitters from vesicles. The neurotransmitters pass across the axon through to the synaptic cleft or synapse, bind to special molecules called receptors and open channels located on the postsynaptic neuron of the target organ or cell.

9. Give an example of a neurotransmitter.
   ✓ Dopamine, serotonin, glutamate, acetylcholine, histamine, noradrenaline, adrenaline are all neurotransmitters.

10. Dopamine is found in the brain. True or false?
    ✓ This is true; dopamine is of one the various neurotransmitters found in the brain. Dopamine helps to control the brain's reward and pleasure centres and helps to regulate movement and emotional responses.

11. If someone has low serotonin levels in their brain, what are the likely health implications?
    ✓ Irritability, depression, hostility and sleep disturbances could occur.

12. To understand how psychotropic medicines work, it is important to understand the theory behind neurotransmitter pathways and mechanisms in the brain. True or false?
    ✓ This is true. The pharmacological effects of drugs used in mental health can enhance or dampen biochemical pathways of neurotransmitters and receptors in the brain. These effects can either provide relief from common symptoms of mental illness, such as hallucinations and disorganised thinking, but also may result in unwanted effects, for example extrapyramidal side effects commonly associated with typical antipsychotic drugs.

13. What are the likely health effects of having low glutamate?
    ✓ A reduction in glutamate (an excitatory neurotransmitter in the brain) can result in mania and hallucinations. Drugs that compete and antagonise the NMDA receptor (glutamate receptor) can induce both positive and negative symptoms in healthy people and people with schizophrenia.

14. In Alzheimer's disease, low acetylcholine neurotransmitter is likely to lead to poor memory.

15. What does CNS stand for?
    ✓ The central nervous system (CNS) is made up of the brain and the spinal cord.

16. What might be the effects of having too much glutamate?
    ✓ Increased levels of glutamate lead to neural death/degeneration, which results in poor memory function/learning.

17. What might be the effects of having too much dopamine?
    ✓ Disorganised thoughts, loose associations, disabling compulsions, tics, stereotypical behaviours and psychosis.

18. Name one excitatory and one inhibitory neurotransmitter.
    ✓ GABA and serotonin.
    ✓ Refer to Table 1.1 under Chapter 1 for other correct options.

19. The genetic contribution of genes has been demonstrated by what type of studies?
✓ The genetic contribution to the aetiology of schizophrenia is significant and has been demonstrated by twin, family and adoption studies. The higher incidence of schizophrenia in the families of patients with schizophrenia has inspired many valuable investigations on the genetic basis of schizophrenia. However, the lack of 100 per cent concordance in monozygotic twins is evidence that the aetiology of schizophrenia is not wholly genetic.

20. What are the clinical uses of lorazepam?
✓ Lorazepam is a short-acting benzodiazepine which can produce a calming effect for the agitated or anxious person and can help to reduce excessive levels of anxiety.

21. There are approximately between <u>30–100</u> neurotransmitter molecule types, with <u>ten</u> of them doing 99 per cent of the work.

22. The loss of motor control and changes in personality may occur when there is a lack of what neurotransmitter?
✓ GABA.

23. Impulses resulting from neurotransmitter transmission travel in the nerve cell may initiate one of many actions inside or outside the brain. Give examples of the actions.
✓ Triggering another nerve impulse.
✓ A muscle contraction.
✓ A glandular secretion.

24. What might be the effects of excess serotonin?
✓ Sedation, if greatly increased, can lead to hallucinations and mania.

25. Give two examples of neurodegenerative conditions.
✓ Parkinson's disease, dementia.

26. What is the relationship between neurotransmitters and vesicles?
✓ Neurotransmitters are situated and released from vesicles. The neurotransmitters pass across the axon through to the synaptic cleft or synapse, bind to special molecules called receptors and open channels located on the postsynaptic neuron of the target organ or cell. The open channels release charged ions into the postsynaptic neuron, which initiates one of the following actions:
✓ Triggering another nerve impulse.
✓ A muscle contraction.
✓ A glandular secretion.

27. What factors should be considered by psychiatrists and mental health nurse prescribers when preparing a prescription of psychotropic drugs?
✓ Side effects of the drugs.
✓ Family history.

✓ Existing physical health conditions.

✓ A patient's concordance to medication.

✓ Lifestyle behaviours, such as smoking, illicit substance use.

✓ Past response to a drug.

✓ Pregnancy.

✓ Polypharmacy.

✓ Drug allergies.

✓ Consideration of other drugs (prescribed or recreational).

28. What does CBT stand for? Give a brief description.

✓ Cognitive behaviour therapy; a talking therapy commonly used in patients presenting with common and severe mental illness that can help to manage problems by changing the way they think and behave. CBT is most frequently used to treat anxiety and depression but can be used to manage other mental and physical health problems.

29. What condition could result from having low dopamine?

✓ Parkinson's disease.

30. In the case scenario about Tom, which drug is responsbile for him experiencing dizziness, light-headedness, drowsiness, headache and muscle stiffness?

✓ Haloperidol.

Chapter 2

1. Briefly describe the dopamine and glutamate hypothesis of schizophrenia.

✓ The dopamine theory suggests that positive and negative symptoms in schizophrenia result from increased and decreased dopamine neurotransmission in the mesolimbic and mesocortical pathways respectively.

✓ The glutamate theory suggests that hypofunction of glutamate and antagonism of NMDA receptors in the brain could contribute to the positive and negative psychotic symptoms reported in schizophrenia.

2. What is the full name of the NMDA receptor and which neurotransmitter is associated with this receptor?

✓ N-Methyl-D-aspartate receptor.

✓ Glutamate.

3. Give two predisposing factors for the incidence of weight gain in the psychiatric population.

✓ Unhealthy lifetsyle behaviours.

✓ Sedentary behaviours.

✓ Pharmacological adverse effects of antipsychotic drugs on the body.

✓ Genes.
✓ Mental illness.

4. Weight gain is an adverse side effect of antipsychotic drugs. True or false?
   ✓ True.

5. What is NMS and what does it stand for?
   ✓ Neuroleptic malignant syndrome (NMS) is a potentially life-threatening, neurological disorder, most often caused by an adverse reaction to neuroleptic or antipsychotic drugs; characterised by symptoms of fever, confusion, muscle rigidity, labile blood pressure, sweating and fast heart rate.

6. Give examples of extrapyramidal side effects.
   ✓ Dystonia (usually develops within four hours following drug administration).
   ✓ Tardive dyskinesia (usually develops within four months following drug administration).
   ✓ Akathisia (usually develops within four days following drug administration).
   ✓ Bradykinesia/parkinsonism (usually develops within four weeks following drug administration).

7. Give an example of a high-potency antipsychotic.
   ✓ Haloperidol, flupentixol, pimozide, risperidone and prochlorperazine.

8. List six best practices that need to be observed when monitoring patients taking clozapine.
   ✓ Cardiac enzymes – troponin to be monitored while on treatment. Myocarditis is the most publicised cardiac complication of clozapine treatment, but cardiomyopathy and pericarditis have also been reported.
   ✓ Full blood counts (FBCs), liver function tests (LFTs), ECG, urea and electrolytes (U&Es) before initiation on clozapine.
   ✓ Baseline blood pressure and pulse every one to three hours during first week of initiation.
   ✓ Monitor leucocytes/neutrophils weekly for first 18 weeks, fortnightly up to one year and monthly after.
   ✓ White cell count must be taken if patient develops a fever, flu-like symptoms, sore throat, rash, unexplained bruising, fatigue, malaise, cough, oral mucosal infections, pyrexia.
   ✓ Traffic light system – green, amber, red usually used by Clozapine Patient Management Services (CPMS) for safe prescribing, administration and monitoring of patients taking clozapine. All patients taking clozapine are centrally registered on this service or a familiar service to promote safety and therapeutic use of this drug in mental health settings.
   Green: when all blood results are within acceptable range.
   Amber: blood results are slightly under required markers (neutrophil and leucocyte count), but not clinically significant to deter continuation on treatment.

Red: when both leucocytes and neutrophils are dangerously low and are clinically significant, or when there is physical health symptomatology related to clozapine treatment in which case the clinical team must stop clozapine immediately.

✓ The amount of clozapine that can be supplied varies depending on a patient's stage of monitoring (weekly, fortnightly, monthly): if on weekly, then the patient will only receive medication for up to seven days, if fortnightly, the patient will be dispensed up to 14 days' worth of clozapine and so forth. This is done for safety reasons around management and monitoring of the haematological effects of clozapine, and so the clinical team must review the patient on clozapine weekly, fortnightly, monthly and at routine planned team review meetings to assess overall progress and recovery.

✓ Clozapine assay (blood plasma levels) may be taken to assess and monitor compliance to drug treatment regimen, and in cases where patients are smokers, the titration dose might have to be adjusted as smoking induces and increases activity of liver enzymes (CPY450) resulting in accelerated breakdown of clozapine, thus reducing clozapine levels. When the patient stops smoking, the clinical team must assess response to treatment and act appropriately to reduce/titrate clozapine to a much lower dose.

✓ Patients who have missed clozapine doses for more than 48 hours will need to have the medicine re-titrated.

✓ If more than three days of clozapine is missed, patients' blood testing frequency may need to change.

9. Give clinical features that may indicate a 'red light' or worrying signs/symptoms when a patient is taking clozapine.
    ✓ Systolic blood pressure less than 100 or greater than 170.
    ✓ Diastolic blood pressure less than 60 or greater than 100.
    ✓ Postural drop of systolic blood pressure greater than 20 mmHg or diastolic blood pressure greater than 10 mmHg.
    ✓ Pulse greater than 100 bpm.
    ✓ Temperature higher than 37.5°C OR lower than 35.5°C.
    ✓ If the patient develops unexplained fever, sore throat and flu-like symptoms usually at commencement of clozapine therapy or during dose changes between intervals.
    ✓ Dangerously low levels of white blood count, leucocyte or neutrophil count.
    ✓ Patient complaining of constipation.

10. What are depot medications?
    ✓ Depot medications are slow-release drug formulations, often used to treat and manage mental disorders such as schizophrenia and psychotic depression.

11. How do depot medications differ from oral antipsychotics?
    ✓ Depot antipsychotics are administered by deep intramuscular injection, usually at intervals of one to four weeks.

12. What is the metabolic syndrome?
    ✓ Metabolic syndrome refers to a cluster of conditions, which when combined increase the risk of CVDs, stroke and heart attacks.

13. What clinical features must be present for metabolic syndrome to be diagnosed?
    ✓ Hyperlipidaemia (raised triglycerides, cholesterol levels).
    ✓ Raised glucose levels.
    ✓ Hypertension.
    ✓ Abdominal obesity.

14. What are the health risks of obesity and how is weight gain related to antipsychotic drugs?
    ✓ Social disengagement.
    ✓ Non-adherence to medication.
    ✓ Increased risk of physical health conditions and mortality.
    ✓ Dyslipidemia.
    ✓ Diabetes.
    ✓ Polycystic ovary syndrome.
    ✓ Hypertension.
    ✓ Respiratory conditions.
    ✓ Osteoarthritis.
    ✓ Depression.
    ✓ Weight gain has been reported with almost every antipsychotic drug used in mental health settings. Clozapine and olanzapine in particular appear to cause significant weight gain, more so than most typical antipsychotics.

15. What are the common management/interventions for patients taking antipsychotic drugs?
    ✓ Monitor blood pressure lying and standing.
    ✓ Monitor pulse, temperature, respirations.
    ✓ Health promotion around unhealthy lifetyle behaviours (smoking, unhealthy diet, sedentary lifestyle).
    ✓ Monitor liver function tests.
    ✓ Monitor urea and electrolytes (U&Es) and creatinine.
    ✓ Monitor FBC.
    ✓ Monitor ECG.
    ✓ Monitor weight and BMI.
    ✓ Monitor adverse effects of psychotropic drugs.
    ✓ Assess and monitor for physical health conditions, diabetes and glucose intolerance.

16. What is the mesocortical pathway and what is its relevance to the pathophysiology of schizophrenia?
    ✓ Negative symptoms (withdrawal or lack of function, blunt affect, lack of motivation, thought disorder) in schizophrenia have been attributed to hypofunction of the dopaminergic neurotransmitter system situated in the mesocortical pathway in the brain.

17. What is the mesolimbic pathway and what is its relevance to the pathophysiology of schizophrenia?
    ✓ It is proposed that excess of dopaminergic action in the mesolimbic pathway results in positive symptoms of schizophrenia (hallucinations in any sensory modality, delusions).

18. What is the tuberoinfundibular pathway and what is its relevance to the pathophysiology of schizophrenia and drug treatment?

✓ Since dopamine acts as a regulatory mechanism for the production of prolactin, by blocking the actions of dopamine, antipsychotic drugs interfere with this pathway, resulting in hyperprolactinaemia (raised prolactin levels in the blood). Monitoring of prolactin may be required in patients showing symptoms of raised prolactine levels, eg erectile dysfunction, enlarged/painful breasts, delayed orgasms and lactation. Offending drugs may need to be stopped or reducing doses may be required.

19. What is the nigrostriatal pathway and what is its relevance to the pathophysiology of schizophrenia and drug treatment?

✓ Antagonism of dopamine by antipsychotic drugs in the nigrostriatal pathway is said to result in extrapyramidal side effects. In the UK, NICE recommends atypical drugs as first-line treatment for psychosis/schizophrenia. Atypical drugs, in comparison to typical drugs, have a lower propensity to induce extrapyramidal side effects, but are linked to a higher incidence of metabolic risk factors, eg obesity, glucose intolerance and dyslipidaemia.

20. Give two examples of tools used in practice to monitor for side effects of psychotropic drugs.

✓ Glasgow antipsychotic side effects scale (GASS) – 22 questions and can be self-administered by the patient.

✓ Liverpool University neuroleptic side effect rating scale (LUNSERS) – 52 questions.

✓ Abnormal involuntary movement scale (AIMS) – 12 items.

21. What are some likely health implications (side effects) of dopamine antagonist drugs like haloperidol?

Adverse side effects associated with haloperidol can include but are not limited to:

✓ Headache, dizziness, spinning sensation.

✓ Drowsiness.

✓ Sleep problems (insomnia).

✓ Feeling restless.

✓ Mild skin rash or itching.

✓ Breast enlargement.

✓ Irregular menstrual periods.

22. Give three examples of typical and atypical drugs and the maximum daily dose ranges.

✓ Typical drugs:

Chlorpromazine (25–1000 mg)

Promazine (100–800 mg)

Trifluoperazine (Stelazine; 10–40 mg)
Haloperidol (2.5–30 mg)
✓ Atypical:
Aripiprazole (5–30 mg)
Clozapine (12.5–900 mg)
Olanzapine (2.5–20 mg)
Quetiapine (25–800 mg)

23. What are anticholinergics and can you give two examples?
✓ Anticholinergic drugs help to reduce and provide relief of some of the extrapy-ramidal side effects caused by dopamine antagonism by antipsychotic drugs. In practice, procyclidine and ophenadrine are commonly used. They both come in three different forms: tablets, liquid and intramascular injection.

24. What is the difference between tardive dyskinesia and dystonia?
✓ Tardive dyskinesia results from chronic administration of antipsychotic drugs, especially typical drug agents. Tardive dyskinesia is the term conventionally used to describe stereotypic, repetitive, abnormal movements of the face, mouth, lips and tongue.
✓ Dystonia is usually an acute reaction, with onset generally one to four hours after drug administration. It clinically manifests as involuntary contractions of the muscles of the head, spine, laryngeal, face and neck muscles. It is very painful and often frightening for the patient.

25. What is agranulocytosis? Which antipsychotic drug is mostly associated with this condition?
✓ Agranulocytosis is a severe and significant reduction in leukocytes (white blood cells), which can be life-threatening due to the high risk of dangerous infection.
✓ Clozapine.

Chapter 3

1. What is the general mechanism of action of antidepressants?
✓ While the precise mode of action of antidepressants remains unclear, a com-mon pharmacological action is suggested to be the enhancement of brain seroto-nin , dopamine and/or noradrenaline neurotransmission.

2. What is serotonin and why is it relevant to the monoamine theory of depression?
✓ Serotonin belongs to a group of neurotransmitters called monoamines.
✓ Among other functions, serotonin inhibits activity and behaviour, increases sleep time, is involved in temperature regulation and controls mood states. It is suggested that MAO enzyme breaks down serotonin (reduces serotonin lev-els in the brain), and this appears to result in clinical symptoms of a depressive pathology.

3. What is your understanding of the term clinical depression?

   ✓ Clinical depression, also known as major depression or major depressive disorder, is marked by severe symptoms of depression (low mood, loss of interest and pleasure, reduced energy, insomnia, excessive feelings of worthlessness and guilt, hopelessness, suicidal thoughts, poor concentration, reduced appetite, anxiety, irritability and weight loss or weight gain) that are persistent and disrupt the person's normal functioning in everyday life.

4. What class of drugs does amitriptyline belong to? State its clinical uses.

   ✓ Amitriptyline is a tricyclic antidepressant,

   ✓ Clinical uses include treatment and management of major depression, chronic pain syndrome, migraine prophylaxis and anxiety.

5. What is serotonin syndrome, and can you describe the symptoms?

   ✓ Serotonin syndrome refers to a cluster of motor, autonomic and mental changes resulting from excess serotonin neurotransmission. Serotonin syndrome can occur when medications that cause high levels of serotonin to accumulate in the body are administered. It often occurs either during dose changes or when adding in new drugs.

   ✓ Symptoms can include: shivering, diarrhoea, muscle rigidity, fever, seizures, confusion, rapid heart rate, high blood pressure, dilated pupils, hyperactivity, tremors, loss of muscle co-ordination or twitching muscles. Severe serotonin syndrome can be fatal if not treated.

6. What is the usual dose range of citalopram and why is it not recommended for doses greater than 40 mg?

   ✓ Recommended daily dose range: 10–40 mg (adults), 10–20 mg (older adults and in patients with poor liver function).

   ✓ Higher doses have been associated with increased risk to cardiovascular health, eg QT interval prolongation, which can lead to arrhythmias.

7. Suicidal thoughts are a potential side effect of antidepressants. True or false?

   ✓ This statement is true; fluoxetine has been associated with increased suicidal ideations in young people.

8. What is St John's Wort?

   ✓ This is a readily available herbal preparation that appears to have antidepressant effects. As it is widely available on the internet and in high-street herbalist stores, co-administration of this herbal drug with pharmacological antidepressants must be avoided to prevent overstimulation of serotonin neurotransmission. In addition, before starting a patient on a pharmacological antidepressant, prescribers need to specifically enquire about any over-the-counter drugs the patient may be taking. Patient education about co-administration with over-the-counter drugs is important.

9. What does SSRI stand for? Give three examples of drugs from this class.
   ✓ Selective serotonin reuptake inhibitor.
   ✓ Citalopram, escitalopram, fluoxetine, paroxetine, sertraline, fluvoxamine.

10. What is tyramine and why is this chemical relevant to patients taking MAOIs?
    ✓ Tyramine is a substance found in common foods such as cheese, yeast extracts, some beers, pickled herring, broad beans, Oxo, Marmite and red wine.
    ✓ MAOIs inhibit the action of MAO enzyme in the presynaptic neuron. This enzyme normally breaks down tyramine and noradrenaline in the body; by inhibiting the MAO enzyme, MAOIs can lead to increased levels of tyramine and noradrenaline in the blood, which can result in cardiovascular abnormalities including hypertensive crises, stroke, and even intracerebral haemorrhage and death.

11. When switching from a SSRI to MAOI, how many days should elapse before starting MAOIs?
    ✓ Five weeks for fluoxetine, two weeks for other SSRIs.

12. List some of the common side effects of SSRIs.
    ✓ Anxiety, drowsiness, insomnia, nervousness, lethargy.
    ✓ Nausea, bloating, diarrhoea.
    ✓ Weight loss, loss of appetite.
    ✓ Sexual dysfunction.

13. What factors should prescribers consider in selection and/or choice of an antidepressant?
    ✓ The nature and degree of clinical symptomatology.
    ✓ Safety in overdose.
    ✓ Previous treatment response to a drug.
    ✓ The drug's side effects profile, interactions with concurrent drugs and physical illness.
    ✓ Patient preference and clinical benefit in cases where there are associated comorbid physical and psychiatric conditions.

14. What cardiovascular adverse effects are associated with TCAs?
    ✓ QT prolongation (for example, amitriptyline, nortriptyline, imipramine).
    ✓ Tachycardia and arrhythmias, especially if there is cardiac conduction delay.
    ✓ The most common serious cardiovascular complication of most TCAs is orthostatic hypotension.

15. Which class of antidepressants is recommended by NICE as a first choice for treatment of moderate to severe major depressive disorder?
    ✓ SSRIs, eg sertraline, citalopram, fluoxetine, paroxetine.

16. Name some of the common foods rich in tyramine.
    ✓ Aged cheeses like cheddar, blue cheese, broad beans, yeast extracts, some beers, pickled herring, Oxo, Marmite and red wine. It is best to avoid consuming these foods/drinks when taking MAOIs.

17. What signs/symptoms may occur if antidepressants are withdrawn abruptly?
     ✓ Anxiety.
     ✓ Electric shock sensations.
     ✓ Fatigue.
     ✓ Flu-like symptoms.
     ✓ Headache.
     ✓ Loss of co-ordination.
     ✓ Muscle spasms.
     ✓ Depression and mood swings.

18. What are the clinical indications of bupropion?
     ✓ Smoking cessation.
     ✓ Major depression (unlicensed).
     ✓ Bipolar disorder (depressive phase).
     ✓ Chronic fatigue syndrome.
     ✓ Lower back pain.

19. What physical health measures might you need to carry out to monitor a patient taking antidepressants?
     ✓ Vital signs – blood pressure, pulse, temperature, respirations.
     ✓ Blood tests – FBCs, U&Es, creatinine, LFTs, lipid/cholesterol tests, glycaemic tests.
     ✓ ECG.
     ✓ Weight, girth measures and BMI.
     ✓ Lifestyle screening – smoking, sedentary behaviour, unhealthy dietary habits.
     ✓ Health screening scales – Becks depression inventory, Generalised Anxiety Disorder-7 (GAD-7), Patient Health Questionnaire-9 (PHQ-9), Mini-Mental State Examination (MMSE) and a Mental State Examination (MSE).

20. All antidepressants could induce mania/hypomanic symptoms in people with bipolar disorder if they are not concurrently taking a mood stabiliser such as lithium.

Chapter 4

1.   What symptoms are commonly associated with dementia?
     ✓ Decline in memory, thinking, comprehension, orientation, language, personality, intellect and behaviour.

2.   Anti-dementia drugs are also known as cognitive enhancers.

3.   Antipsychotics and benzodiazepines can be adjunct treatment options to manage which symptoms of dementia?

✓ Behavioural and psychological symptoms such as: apathy, wandering, appetite disturbance, irritability, agitation, aggression, sleep disturbance, depression, anxiety, delusions, disinhibition and hallucinations.

✓ The use of medication for behavioural management is controversial; therefore the use of antipsychotics and benzodiazepines should be reviewed regularly to assess effectiveness, and whether it can be reduced or stopped.

4. Name two classes of drugs used to manage symptoms related to dementia.
    ✓ Acetylcholinesterase inhibitors.
    ✓ NMDA receptor antagonist.

5. What is the mechanism of action of acetylcholinesterase inhibitors?
    ✓ Acetylcholinesterase inhibitors reduce the breakdown of acetylcholine by the enzyme acetylcholinesterase; this action increases central acetylcholine neurotransmission.

6. What is the mechanism of action of memantine?
    ✓ Hyper-function of glutamate on NMDA receptors results in nerve cell damage. Memantine is a NMDA receptor antagonist and therefore blocks these neurotoxic consequences of glutamate overstimulation. Although memantine does not target acetylcholine, it is thought to have neuroprotective effects on cholinergic nerve cells via its actions of blocking the excessive effects on glutamate on NMDA receptors.

7. What is polypharmacy and of what relevance is this to an older patient?
    ✓ Polypharmacy is the concurrent use of five or more medications; this is more common in the older person as they often have multiple physical health co-morbidities. Due to age-related physiological changes that can alter the way in which drugs are handled by the body of the older person, polypharmacy increases the risk of adverse drug reactions and interactions, such as agitation, confusion and risk of falls.

8. Give examples of acetylcholinesterase inhibitors.
    ✓ Rivastigmine, donepezil, galantamine.

9. Describe the side effects associated with memantine.
    ✓ Fatigue.
    ✓ Headache.
    ✓ Dizziness.
    ✓ Constipation.
    ✓ Somnolence.
    ✓ Hypertension.
    ✓ Vomiting.
    ✓ Anxiety.
    ✓ Hallucinations.

10. Describe side effects associated with cholinesterase inhibitors.
   ✓ Nausea, vomiting.
   ✓ Diarrhoea.
   ✓ Vertigo, dizziness, fainting.
   ✓ Insomnia, nightmares.
   ✓ Agitation.
   ✓ Headache.
   ✓ Muscle cramps.
   ✓ Tremors.
   ✓ Fatigue.
   ✓ Weight loss.

11. What is acetylcholine?
   ✓ Acetylcholine is a neurotransmitter; its main functions are to stimulate muscles and aid in memory function.

12. What is glutamate?
   ✓ Glutamate is a major excitatory neurotransmitter involved in functions such as metabolic energy production, neural communication, memory formation, learning, thinking and regulation.

13. Outline routine physical health checks/tests that should be conducted in older patients.
   ✓ FBC.
   ✓ Urea, electrolytes and creatinine level.
   ✓ CRP.
   ✓ LFTs.
   ✓ TFTs.
   ✓ Vitamin B12 and folate levels.
   ✓ Vitamin D, calcium and bone profile.
   ✓ Food and fluid monitoring.
   ✓ BMI and weight measures.
   ✓ Memory testing.
   ✓ Screening for depression, lifestyle factors (smoking, alcohol).
   ✓ Blood pressure, pulse, temperature measures.

14. Name four drug groups commonly involved in drug interactions.
   ✓ Cardiovascular agents.
   ✓ Antibiotics.
   ✓ Diuretics.
   ✓ Anticoagulants.
   ✓ Hypoglycaemic drugs.
   ✓ Steroids.
   ✓ Opioids.
   ✓ Anticholinergics.
   ✓ Benzodiazepines.
   ✓ Non-steroidal anti-inflammatory drugs (NSAIDs).

15. What anti-dementia drug is available in the form of patches?
✓ Rivastigmine.

16. What anti-dementia drug is available in the form of orodispersible tablets?
✓ Donepezil.

17. Generally speaking, the <u>more</u> drugs a patient takes, the <u>greater the risk</u> of adverse reactions and drug interactions.

18. Memantine is licensed for treatment and management of <u>moderate to severe behavioural and psychological symptoms of</u> Alzheimer's disease.

19. Cholinesterase inhibitors often cure the symptoms of Alzheimer's disease. True or false?
✓ False.
✓ Acetylcholinesterase inhibitors may help to treat the symptoms of Alzheimer's disease, but are not a cure – there is no evidence that these drugs can stop or reverse the process of nerve cell loss that causes Alzheimer's disease.

20. What drugs does NICE recommend for the management of mild to moderate symptoms of Alzheimer's disease?
✓ Donepezil.
✓ Galantamine.
✓ Rivastigmine.

21. What risks are associated with the use of antipsychotics in patients with dementia?
✓ The use of antipsychotics could be linked to further deterioration in cognitive function and increased morbidity and mortality. Older patients with dementia are particularly vulnerable to extrapyramidal, anticholinergic and cardiac side effects of antipsychotic drugs.

22. Give three examples of drug classes that may interact with cholinesterase inhibitors.
✓ Antidepressants
✓ Anti-arrhythmia
✓ Antihistamines

23. Is there evidence that cholinesterase inhibitors can stop or reverse the process of nerve cell loss that causes Alzheimer's disease?
✓ No. So far, there is no scientific evidence to support this claim.

24. What is the indication for use of antidepressants in patients with Alzheimer's disease?
✓ Depression is often poorly diagnosed/underdiagnosed in older patients with Alzheimer's disease; antidepressants could be used as additional pharmacotherapy to counter clinical symptoms of depression in this vulnerable patient group.

25. Name three different types of dementia.
    ✓ Alzheimer's disease.
    ✓ Dementia with Lewy bodies.
    ✓ Dementia in Parkinson's disease.
    ✓ Vascular dementia.
    ✓ Mixed dementia (Alzheimer's disease and vascular dementia).

Chapter 5

1. Name the common symptoms reported by patients with mania.
    ✓ Elated mood.
    ✓ Overactivity.
    ✓ Pressure of speech.
    ✓ Disturbed/reduced need for sleep.
    ✓ Increased speed of thought.
    ✓ Poor concetration.
    ✓ Irritability.
    ✓ Social disinhibition.
    ✓ Hallucinations.
    ✓ Mood-congruent delusions, as well as unrealistic, extravagant and grandiose ideas.

2. Is breastfeeding recommended in women on lithium therapy for bipolar disorder?
    ✓ No. Lithium is present in breast milk and carries risk of toxicity for the infant.
    ✓ Similarly, in pregnancy, lithium treatment is associated with an increased risk of cardiac foetal abnormalities.

3. What checks should be conducted before initiating lithium therapy?
    ✓ FBCs, U&Es, serum creatinine, urinalysis, TFTs, eGFR, LFTs, calcium levels, baseline BMI, blood pressure, pulse and an ECG.

4. Why is monitoring serum lithium concentration important in patients?
    ✓ Lithium plasma levels are useful in determining whether the patient is receiving the optimum dose of lithium, ie are the lithium levels within the desired therapeutic range?
    ✓ Provides an indication of patient's drug adherence.
    ✓ Serum drug monitoring allows for assessment of mild lithium toxicity levels or severe toxicity levels, which would then prompt management actions/interventions accordingly.

5. Can you give examples of symptoms associated with lithium toxicity?
    ✓ Muscle weakness.
    ✓ Drowsiness.
    ✓ Ataxia.

✓ Coarse tremors.

✓ Dysarthria.

✓ Muscle twitching.

✓ Cardiac arrhythmias.

✓ Increased disorientation and confusion.

✓ Seizures.

✓ Acute renal failure.

✓ Coma, and ultimately death.

6. State the target serum lithium concentration range, within which lithium is at safe and effective levels?

   ✓ 0.4–1.0 mmol/L.

7. What mood stabiliser does NICE recommend as first-line management of acute mania and bipolar disorder for patients in secondary care?

   ✓ Lithium.

8. Antipsychotics are routinely used solely or in combination with mood stabilisers in the treatment and management of bipolar disorder. True or false?

   ✓ True.

9. What risks are associated with the use of antidepressants in bipolar disorder?

   ✓ Antidepressant use, without a concomitant mood stabiliser, in patients with bipolar disorder is associated with a significantly increased risk for subsequent manic episodes and rapid cycling.

10. What is a teratogen?

    ✓ An agent/drug (prescribed or recreational) that can cause malformation/abnormality in a developing embryo.

11. Carbamazepine and clozapine are both known to cause agranulocytosis. What does this term mean?

    ✓ Both drugs are associated with a high risk of inducing blood disorders.

    ✓ Agranulocytosis is a potentially life-threatening condition, characterised by a dangerously low white blood cell count (most commonly of neutrophils) and so the patient is at increased vulnerability to infection.

12. Give examples of three antipsychotic drugs that may be used in the management of bipolar disorder.

    ✓ Olanzapine, risperidone, quetiapine, aripiprazole, asenapine.

13. What does the abbreviation 'FBC' stand for and what does this test measure?

    ✓ Full blood count – blood test that checks levels of red blood cells, white blood cells and platelets.

14. Does lithium have a narrow or a wide therapeutic index? What does this mean for you as a health professional?

 ✓ Lithium has a narrow therapeutic index which means there are few differences between therapeutic and toxic doses. Therefore, regular drug plasma monitoring is mandatory for all patients on lithium to ensure levels are within the safe and effective therapeutic range (0.4–1.0mmol/L) and to be able to quickly identify patients with potentially toxic levels of the drug.

15. What are some symptoms of mild to moderate lithium toxicity?

 ✓ Anorexia.

 ✓ Vomiting.

 ✓ Nausea.

 ✓ Diarrhoea.

 ✓ Polyuria.

 ✓ Muscle weakness and twitching.

 ✓ Drowsiness.

 ✓ Ataxia.

 ✓ Dysarthria.

 ✓ Coarse tremors.

16. Name a mood stabiliser which is a potent cytochrome P450 enzyme inducer.

 ✓ Carbamazepine.

17. Why is it important for doctors and nurses to always ask about a patient's past and current medication history?

 ✓ This is a vital aspect of the health assessment which will provide important information to the clinician about the patient.

 ✓ Past medication history will inform the health professional about previous treatment response to a drug, side effects, adverse drug reactions and allergies.

 ✓ Asking about a patient's past and current medication history can help the clinician to understand the patient's health beliefs, values and concerns about medications, especially to address issues around non-concordance.

 ✓ Accurate and comprehensive current medication history provides important information that will inform prescribing decisions in terms of avoiding drug interactions and provides insight into a patient's other co-morbidities. A full drug history includes all prescribed medications, medications bought over-the-counter or online and herbal drugs and includes information about other lifestyle activities that may influence prescribing decisions, eg recreational drug use, smoking and alcohol use.

18. Teratogenicity means that lithium and carbamazepine should be avoided in <u>pregnancy</u>.

19. What are the common side effects associated with the use of carbamazepine and sodium valproate?
    ✓ Sedation.
    ✓ Headache.
    ✓ Hyponatraemia.
    ✓ Constipation or diarrhoea.
    ✓ Nausea.
    ✓ Oedema.
    ✓ Vomiting.

20. Can sodium valproate be prescribed to patients with liver dysfunction?
    ✓ Sodium valproate has been associated with causing hepatotoxicity as well as thrombocytopenia at high doses. As such, liver function tests and FBCs should be tested every 6–12 months. Hence, sodium valproate should be avoided or used with caution in patients with liver disease.

21. What worrying symptoms may be present in a patient on carbamazepine with a low WBC count?
    ✓ Paleness of the skin.
    ✓ Bleeding.
    ✓ Mouth ulcers.
    ✓ Weakness.
    ✓ Fever.
    ✓ Any signs of infections.
    ✓ Sore throat.
    ✓ Cough.
    ✓ Bruising easily.
    ✓ Vomiting.
    ✓ Abdominal pain.

22. What medical condition(s) is valproic acid indicated for?
    ✓ Valproic acid is approved for the management of epilepsy while sodium and semi-sodium valproate are approved for the treatment and management of mania.

23. What is the usual daily dose range of sodium valproate?
    ✓ 750–2000 mg

24. Psychotic symptoms are common in patients with bipolar disorder. True or false?
    ✓ True.

25. Why should prescribers avoid withdrawing lithium suddenly in patients with bipolar disorder?
    ✓ If abruptly stopped, this could increase the risk of relapse and lead to re-occurrence of symptoms in the patient.

Chapter 6

1. What are some of the clinical uses of benzodiazepines?
    ✓ Anxiolytic – used in the treatment of severe anxiety.
    ✓ Hypnotic – used in the treatment of insomnia or for sedation.
    ✓ Anticonvulsant – used in the treatment of epilepsy and seizures.
    ✓ Muscle-relaxant – used in the treatment of muscle spasms or acute dystonia.

2. It is common to find benzodiazepines co-administered with an antipsychotic drug.
    True or false?
    ✓ True.

3. What is drug half-life? What is drug potency?
    ✓ The half-life of a drug is how long it takes for the body to eliminate half of the
    dose of that drug from the bloodstream.
    ✓ Drug potency is how strong a drug is and relates to the amount of drug needed
    to achieve a specific effect.

4. Give an example of a benzodiazepine with a long half-life and one with a short/inter-
    mediate half-life.
    ✓ Long-acting benzodiazepines: diazepam, clonazepam, chlordiazepoxide,
    clobazam, flurazepam, nitrazepam.
    ✓ Short/intermediate-acting benzodiazepines: lorazepam, oxazepam, temaz-
    epam, loprazolam.

5. Give examples of six different drugs, from at least three different classes, that are
    licensed for the treatment of anxiety in the UK.
    ✓ Benzodiazepines – oxazepam, lorazepam, diazepam, chlordiazepoxide,
    clobazam, clonazepam.
    ✓ Non-benzodiazepine anxiolytic – buspirone.
    ✓ Antidepressants – SSRIs (eg sertraline), TCAs (eg nortriptyline), venlafaxine,
    trazodone.
    ✓ Atypical anticonvulsant – pregabalin.
    ✓ Typical antipsychotic – trifluoperazine.
    ✓ Beta blockers – propranolol, oxprenolol.

6. What are the major clinical concerns and issues related to prolonged use of anxiolyt-
    ics and hypnotics?
    ✓ The use of both benzodiazepines and hypnotics in the treatment and man-
    agement of anxiety and insomnia is limited by the increased risk for these
    drugs to cause tolerability and dependence (both physical and psychological).
    Withdrawal effects can occur upon stopping the drug, especially after prolonged
    administration.

7. What are the clinical manifestations of a paradoxical reaction to benzodiazepines and which groups of people are mostly at risk?

    ✓ This extreme reaction is usually marked by agitated delirium with emotional lability, hostility, aggression, restlessness, over-excitement, increased rate of speech and anti-social acts.

    ✓ Risk factors for paradoxical reactions include psychiatric comorbidity, the elderly, learning disability, neurological disorders or CNS degenerative disease and alcoholism.

8. Barbiturates are commonly used in clinical practice for the treatment of anxiety disorders in the UK. True or false? What is the rationale for your answer?

    ✓ False.

    ✓ Tolerance to barbiturates occurs more rapidly compared to benzodiazepines, physical dependency may even occur at very small doses and these drugs have far more side effects and drug interactions than benzodiazepines. They are more dangerous in overdose and for these reasons, benzodiazepines have replaced barbiturates as hypnotics and sedatives of choice. However, barbiturates are still sometimes used for general anaesthesia in surgery and in the treatment of epilepsy.

9. What are the symptoms of benzodiazepine withdrawal?

    ✓ Increased anxiety.

    ✓ Insomnia.

    ✓ Aching limbs.

    ✓ Nausea.

    ✓ Nervousness, restlessness.

    ✓ Irritability.

    ✓ Fatigue.

    ✓ Delirium.

    ✓ Tremors.

    ✓ Depression.

10. Benzodiazepines with <u>short</u> half-lives are associated with more acute and intense withdrawal symptoms compared to benzodiazepines with <u>long</u> half-lives.

11. In which organ of the body are drugs often converted into metabolites?

    ✓ Liver.

12. What is the main inhibitory neurotransmitter in the brain?

    ✓ GABA.

13. Give three examples of non-benzodiazepine hypnotics.

    ✓ Z-drugs – zopiclone, zolpidem, zaleplon.

    ✓ Promethazine.

    ✓ Chloral hydrate.

    ✓ Melatonin.

14. What is the name of the receptor site for Z-drugs?
    ✓ Benzodiazepine binding site of GABA-A receptors.
    ✓ Z-drugs drugs are GABA agonists and work in a similar way to the benzodiazepine drugs inside the brain at the GABAergic receptor site but have a different chemical structure than benzodiazepines.

15. Name the antihistamine drug that may be used in the management of insomnia. What are the common side effects associated with this drug?
    ✓ Promethazine.
    ✓ Common side effects include: dizziness, tinnitus, ataxia, blurred vision, restlessness, dry mouth, headaches, skin rashes, urinary retention, constipation.

16. List three differences between buspirone and benzodiazepines.
    ✓ Benzodiazepines usually have rapid onset, while buspirone has a delayed onset.
    ✓ Benzodiazepines induce sedation, whereas buspirone tends to not induce sedation.
    ✓ Benzodiazepines can cause dependency and withdrawal symptoms, whereas buspirone is not addictive.
    ✓ The pharmacokinetics of benzodiazepines, but not buspirone, change with age.
    ✓ Benzodiazepines, but not buspirone, are associated with impaired performance.
    ✓ Benzodiazepines, but not buspirone, are known to cause drug interactions with other CNS depressants.
    ✓ Benzodiazepines cause significant additive CNS depressant effects with alcohol; buspirone causes minimal additive CNS depressant effects with alcohol.
    ✓ Benzodiazepines, but not buspirone, are known to cause drug interactions with other CNS depressants.
    ✓ Benzodiazepines, but not buspirone, are associated with falls in the elderly.

17. Give two examples of beta blockers. What are the clinical benefits of using beta blockers in patients with severe anxiety?
    ✓ Propranolol and oxprenolol.
    ✓ Beta blockers are clinically useful in managing somatic symptoms related to anxiety (palpitations, tremor, sweating) but do not have any clinical effect on the psychological symptoms of anxiety.

18. Name an antipsychotic drug that is also licensed for use in severe anxiety in the UK.
    ✓ Trifluoperazine.
    ✓ This typical antipsychotic drug, which may be used to treat schizophrenia and psychosis, is also indicated for the management of severe anxiety at lower doses

19. What is the usual daily dose range of diazepam and lorazepam?
    ✓ Diazepam: 2–30 mg daily.
    ✓ Lorazepam: 0.5–4 mg daily.

20. What is the name of the drug that can be given (with caution) to reverse the effects of benzodiazepines?
    ✓ Flumazenil – a selective benzodiazepine receptor antagonist.

Glossary

Abdominal obesity

Also known as central obesity; is when excessive abdominal fat around the stomach and abdomen builds up to the extent that it is likely to have a negative impact on health. People with central obesity are at a high risk of developing diabetes, kidney disease, hypertension, dyslipidaemia and cardiovascular disease.

Acetylcholinesterase inhibitor

A drug that increases the levels of neurotransmitter acetylcholine by inhibiting the actions of acetylcholinesterase (an enzyme that breaks down acetylcholine). These drugs are used in the treatment of dementia.

Action potential

The alteration in electrical charge linked to the passage of an impulse along the membrane of a muscle cell or nerve cell.

Affective disorders

This is a term used to describe a group of mental disorders characterised by changes in mood.

Agonist

A drug or ligand that produces a biological response by binding to and activating a receptor.

Agranulocytosis

A potentially life-threatening condition; a severe and acute reduction in granulocytes (white blood cells – basophils, eosinophils and neutrophil) as an extreme reaction to a drug, resulting in the patient being at a dangerously high risk of infection. Clozapine and Carbamazepine are two examples of drugs that have been known to cause agranulocytosis.

Allergy

Allergies/allergic diseases are various conditions caused by hypersensitivity of the immune system to something (allergen) in the environment or a drug that usually causes little or no problem in most people.

Amyloid cascade theory

This theory proposes that excessive accumulation of a peptide called beta-amyloid in the brain is the key event in the pathophysiology of Alzheimer's disease. This accumulation of beta-amyloid plaques sets in motion a series of events which result in the death of nerve cells and subsequently leads to Alzheimer's disease.

Angioedema	A potentially life-threatening reaction resulting in sudden swelling of the face, neck, lips, tongue, throat, hands, feet, lips or genitals. Angioedema is usually triggered by an allergic reaction to a food, drug or insect bite.
Antagonist (drug)	A drug or ligand that blocks or dampens a biological response by binding to and blocking a receptor (rather than activating it like an agonist).
Anticholinergic drugs	A drug or substance that blocks the actions of the neurotransmitter acetylcholine in the parasympathetic nervous system.
Anticonvulsants	A drug used mainly to prevent or reduce epileptic fits and other seizures. Some anticonvulsants like sodium valproate and carbamazepine are also used to treat and manage patients with bipolar disorder.
Arrhythmias	This term refers to abnormal heart rhythms.
Ataxia	Lack of co-ordination of muscle action, particularly when walking or holding objects.
Barbiturates	A class of sedative and sleep-inducing drugs obtained from barbituric acid.
Benzodiazepines	A class of drugs that act as tranquilisers; used in the treatment and management of moderate to severe anxiety.
Biotransformation	A process by which organic compounds (typically drugs) are chemically changed from one form to another within the body, usually through the action of enzymes.
Bipolar disorder	Bipolar disorder is a common debilitating psychiatric illness characterised by repeated episodes of mania, hypomania or depression with complete inter-episode recovery.
Blood-brain barrier	The blood-brain barrier (BBB) is a highly selective semipermeable membrane barrier that separates the circulating blood from the brain tissues. It protects the brain from harmful substances that may enter the bloodstream.
Bradykinesia	Abnormally slow body movement. Bradykinesia is a key feature of parkinsonism and is a commonly reported side effect in patients taking antipsychotic drugs.
Cardiac enzymes	These are molecules released into blood circulation because of injury or damage to the heart muscle. Blood

tests can detect abnormally high levels of cardiac enzymes (eg troponin, creatine kinase, myoglobin) and are used in the diagnosis of conditions such as myocardial infarction (heart attack) and myocarditis (inflammation of heart muscle).

Cardiomyopathy

Refers to diseases of the heart muscle, where it becomes abnormally enlarged, thick or rigid.

Cardiotoxicity

A condition where there is damage to the heart muscle by harmful chemicals or drugs, and as a result the heart becomes weaker and may be unable to pump blood effectively.

Clozapine

An atypical antipsychotic drug which is mainly used in the treatment of schizophrenia that does not improve after trials of other antipsychotic medications.

Cognitive Behavioural Therapy (CBT)

A psychosocial intervention that uses a systematic approach and goal-oriented therapy to address dysfunctional thoughts, emotions and behaviours. CBT is commonly used to treat anxiety and depression, but can be beneficial for many other mental and physical health problems.

Cytochrome P450 (CYP) enzymes

CYP enzymes, primarily located in the liver, are an essential group of enzymes involved in the metabolism of drugs or other substances. Most drugs are deactivated by CYPs and transformed into a form that is readily eliminated from the body. Other drugs are bioactivated by CYPs to form their active compounds. There are up to 60 CYP enzymes in humans and the majority of these play a central role in drug metabolism.

Dementia

An umbrella term for a range of progressive disorders of the brain affecting mental processes and functioning, giving rise to symptoms that include memory loss and difficulties with thinking, problem solving, language and/or behaviour. Dementia is diagnosed when these symptoms are severe enough to affect the person's activities of daily living. There are many different types of dementia including: Alzheimer's disease, vascular dementia, and dementia with Lewy bodies.

Diabetes mellitus

A medical condition in which the body's ability to produce or respond to the insulin hormone is impaired, resulting in elevated levels of glucose in the blood.

Diabetes insipidus	An uncommon disorder characterised by intense thirst (polydipsia) and excretion of large amounts of urine (polyuria). It can be caused by damage to the brain (central diabetes insipidus) or may be due to a problem with the kidneys (nephrogenic).
DNA (deoxyribonucleic acid)	DNA is a self-replicating molecule, containing genetic information, and is present in nearly all living organisms as the main constituent of chromosomes.
Dopamine hypothesis of schizophrenia	The dopamine theory suggests that positive and negative symptoms in schizophrenia result from increased and decreased dopamine neurotransmission in the mesolimbic and mesocortical pathways respectively.
Drug dependence	Also known as substance dependence; develops from repeated dosing or administration such that the person experiences physical withdrawal symptoms upon stopping or withdrawing the agent or drug.
Drug interaction	This is the modification of the activity of a drug by another drug or substance, and can be beneficial or harmful.
Drug tolerance	When a patient develops a diminished response to a drug/substance as a result of frequent use, such that the patient requires increasing doses of the drug over time to achieve the same effect.
Dual diagnosis	The term given to a patient who has a mental illness and a comorbid substance abuse problem. These patients have complex needs and require a lot of community support. Co-occurring and complex needs are terms usually used to refer to dual diagnosis patients.
Dyslipidaemia	An abnormal amount of lipids (fat) in the blood; namely high levels of triglycerides, total cholesterol or low-density lipoprotein (LDL) cholesterol, and/or low levels of high-density lipoprotein (HDL) cholesterol.
Dyspnoea	A state in which the person experiences shortness of breath or difficulty breathing.
Enzyme inducer	A type of drug that increases the metabolic activity of an enzyme (typically those involved in drug metabolism, ie cytochrome P450 enzymes), usually resulting in a decrease in the effect of other drugs. Carbamazepine is an example of a drug that is an enzyme inducer.

Enzyme inhibitor	A type of drug that decreases the metabolic activity of an enzyme (typically those involved in drug metabolism, ie cytochrome P450 enzymes), usually resulting in an increase in the effect of other drugs, and can lead to drug toxicity. Paroxetine is an example of a drug that is an enzyme inhibitor, as well as some antibiotics such as erythromycin or ciprofloxacin.
Enzymes	Proteins that act as biological catalysts within cells; they increase the rate at which chemical reactions occur in the body.
Extrapyramidal side effects (EPS)	These are drug-induced movement disorders; physical symptoms resulting from adverse effects of dopamine antagonist agents (principally antipsychotic drugs) blocking dopamine transmission in the nervous system. EPS includes: dystonia, akathisia, parkinsonism and tardive dyskinesia.
GABA (gamma-aminobutyric acid)	The main inhibitory neurotransmitter in the brain; GABA receptors are widely situated throughout cortical and subcortical regions of the brain.
Glutamate hypothesis of schizophrenia	The glutamate theory suggests that hypofunction of glutamate and antagonism of N-methyl-D-aspartate (NMDA) receptors in the brain could contribute to the positive and negative psychotic symptoms reported in schizophrenia.
Half-life	The time it takes for the concentration of a drug in the bloodstream to reduce by half.
Hallucinations	Profound distortions in a person's perception of reality in the context of visual, auditory, tactile and/or olfactory sensory modalities.
Hepatotoxicity	Refers to a drug or chemical that causes adverse effects and damage to the liver.
Hypoglycaemia	Low blood glucose levels.
Hyponatraemia	Low levels of sodium in the blood.
Hypothyroidism	Abnormally low production of thyroid hormone by the thyroid gland; also commonly referred to as 'underactive thyroid'.
Hyperlipidaemia	High levels of lipids (fats, triglycerides and/or cholesterol) in the blood.

Hyperprolactinaemia	Abnormally high levels of prolactin hormone in the blood.
Hypertension	Abnormally high blood pressure.
Limbic system	A complex system of networks in the brain, connecting several subcortical structures associated with instinct, mood and memory. The limbic system controls the basic emotions (fear, pleasure, anger) and drives hunger, sex and dominance.
Lithium	A mood stabilising drug commonly used in the treatment and management of bipolar disorder.
Lorazepam	An intermediate-acting benzodiazepine used in the management of anxiety disorders, insomnia, active seizures and for sedation.
Macroglossia	A medical term used to refer to the severe enlargement of the tongue, which can cause difficulties with breathing, speaking and eating.
Memantine	A NMDA (glutamate) receptor antagonist used in the management of moderate to severe dementia.
Metabolic syndrome	Also known as syndrome X or dysmetabolic syndrome; a cluster of conditions which when combined increase the risk of cardiovascular diseases, stroke and heart attacks. The defining medical conditions that are present in the metabolic syndrome are: abdominal obesity, high blood pressure, high glucose levels and dyslipidaemia or risk factors.
Metabolites	These substances are intermediate products of metabolic reactions, broken down by various enzymes that naturally occur within cells.
Mixed states	In bipolar disorder, mixed states refer to when manic and depressive symptoms are experienced together.
Monoamine hypothesis of depression	This theory postulates that hypofunction in the neurotransmitter pathways of serotonin, noradrenaline and dopamine could reflect the symptoms seen in depression.
Myocarditis	A medical condition where the heart muscle becomes inflamed.

Neuroleptic malignant syndrome (NMS)

A potentially life-threatening neurological disorder, most often caused by an adverse reaction to antipsychotic drugs, characterised by symptoms of fever, confusion, muscle rigidity, labile blood pressure, sweating and fast heart rate.

Neuroleptics

Another term for antipsychotic drugs; a class of drugs used to treat schizophrenia and other psychotic disorders.

Neuron

A neuron or nerve cell is a basic structure of the nervous system; a specialised cell capable of transmitting nerve impulses.

Neurotransmitter

A chemical by which a neuron communicates with another neuron, or with a muscle or gland.

Neutropenia

A condition of abnormally low levels of neutrophils, leading to increased susceptibility to infection.

Neutrophils

A type of white blood cell that attacks bacteria and other organisms when they invade the body, and so help to fight infection.

Oculogyric crisis

This is a type of dystonic adverse reaction to a drug (eg antipsychotics), characterised by a prolonged involuntary upward deviation of the eyes.

Off-label/unlicensed prescribing

This refers to the prescription of a drug outside the terms of its license (eg for a condition other than which it has been officially approved for). In cases of off-label/unlicensed prescribing, the healthcare professional judges the particular prescription to be in the best interests of the patient on the basis of available evidence.

Orthostatic hypotension

Also known as postural hypotension; refers to an abnormal drop in blood pressure that occurs when the person stands up after a period of sitting or lying down. Clozapine, risperidone and quetiapine are examples of atypical antipsychotics that can cause orthostatic hypotension.

Palpitations

Refers to when a person's heartbeat suddenly becomes more noticeable; the person may feel that their heart is beating very fast, fluttering, pounding or beating irregularly.

Panic disorder

A mental condition and anxiety disorder that causes the patient to have recurrent unexpected panic attacks. Panic attacks are sudden periods of intense fear, with accompanying symptoms of: breathlessness, palpitations, sweating, shaking, dizziness, chest pain, numbness/tingling in the hands or a feeling that something terrible is going to happen.

Paralytic ileus

A medical term describing the obstruction of the intestine (gut) due to paralysis of the intestinal muscles; food does not pass through the intestine properly, leading to bloating, blockage, constipation and vomiting.

Pharmacotherapy

The use of pharmaceutical products to treat and manage health conditions, as opposed to surgical treatments or psychological therapies.

Polycystic ovary syndrome (PCOS)

This medical condition is a cluster of symptoms resulting from elevated androgens (male hormones) in women. Symptoms include: irregular menstrual periods, excess body and facial hair, acne, weight gain and difficulty getting pregnant. Women with PCOS often have enlarged ovaries with many large fluid-filled sacs, which fail to regularly release eggs.

Porphyria

Refers to a group of rare genetic disorders that result from a build-up of substances known as porphyrins in the body, which can lead to nerve or skin problems. Some drugs (eg carbamazepine, amitriptyline) can trigger an acute porphyria attack, characterised by: abdominal pain, chest pain, vomiting, confusion, fever, tachycardia and hypertension.

Prophylaxis

Refers to treatment or action taken to prevent a disease.

Psychoactive

A term used to refer to drugs or compounds that can lead to a profound distortion in a person's reality, behaviour and/or emotional state.

Psychotherapy

The use of non-pharmacological interventions to treat and manage health conditions. Examples include: cognitive behavioural therapy (CBT), interpersonal therapy, family therapy and psychoanalysis.

Psychotropic drugs

A range of pharmaceutical products commonly used in the treatment and management of mental disorders.

QTc prolongation

This is seen as an abnormality on ECG and is a surrogate marker for the risk of developing torsades de pointes (TdP). Patients can present with syncope, palpitations, seizures or cardiac arrest. Many drugs can cause QTc prolongation, including some antipsychotics (eg haloperidol, chlorpromazine) and some antidepressants (eg amitriptyline, imipramine).

Rapid cycling

In bipolar disorder, rapid cycling refers to the occurrence of four or more episodes of mania, hypomania or depression within one year.

Rapid tranquillisation (RT)

The process of administering medication to a person often in an emergency who is behaviourally agitated and, in some cases, exhibiting aggressive behaviour posing a risk to themselves and/or others. The purpose and aim of giving the drug is to calm the person quickly and mitigate the risk of aggression and/or violence to themselves and/or others.

Schizophrenia

Eugene Bleuer in 1911 used the term schizophrenia to describe a mental disorder associated with slow progressive deterioration of a person's personality and affect, and which manifests through profound distortions in feelings, thoughts and conduct, and a propensity to withdraw from reality.

Sedation

The act or process of calming following the administration of a drug.

Serotonin (5-hydroxytryptamine, 5-HT)

This is a monoamine neurotransmitter, considered a natural mood stabiliser; serotonin helps in sleeping, eating, mood regulation and digestive processes.

St John's Wort

This is a common and popular non-prescription (over-the-counter) herbal remedy for mild depression that contains the active ingredient Hypericum perforatum.

Suicide

This is a wilful, self-inflicted act that results in the taking of one's own life.

Syncope

Also referred to as fainting; a temporary loss of consciousness, usually caused by a fall in blood pressure or irregular heart rhythm that results in a brief reduction of blood supply to the brain.

Tachycardia

An abnormally fast heart rate.

Tachypnoea

Abnormally fast and shallow breathing.

Teratogen A drug, agent or factor that can cause malformation in a developing embryo.

Therapeutic index The therapeutic index of a drug is a comparison of the dose of the drug that causes the desired therapeutic effect with the dose of the drug that causes serious side effects and toxicity. In drugs that have a narrow therapeutic index (eg lithium) there is little difference between therapeutic and toxic doses. Sometimes, the similar term of 'therapeutic window' is used, which refers to the range of doses of the drug that produces the desired therapeutic response without causing any significant adverse effects in patients.

Thyroid dysfunction A medical condition that affects the function of the thyroid gland, such that it produces abnormally high or abnormally low levels of thyroxine hormone.

Torsades de pointes (TdP) A rare type of arrhythmia characterised by ventricular tachycardia, which manifests as a fast heartbeat, dizziness, fainting and can potentially be life-threatening.

Tricyclic antidepressants (TCAs) First discovered in the 1950s, tricyclics are a group of antidepressants used in the management of major depressive disorder.

Tyramine This is a substance found naturally in some foods. It is especially found in aged and fermented foods, for example: aged cheeses, yeast extracts, red wine, some beers, smoked fish, broad beans, Oxo and Marmite. Prescribers and patients need to be aware of the dangerous potential for interaction between monoamine oxidase inhibitors (a class of antidepressant) and high dietary intake of tyramine, which can result in cardiovascular abnormalities including hypertensive crises, stroke, and even intracerebral haemorrhage and death.

Withdrawal symptoms A group of symptoms, of variable degree of severity, which occur on stopping or reducing the use of a psychoactive substance that has been taken repeatedly, usually for a prolonged period and/ or in high doses.

References

Abi-Dargham, A and Laruelle, M (2005) Mechanisms of Action of Second Generation Antipsychotic Drugs in Schizophrenia: Insights from Brain Imaging Studies. *European Psychiatry*, 20(1): 15–27.

Action on Smoking and Health (2018) Fact Sheet: Smoking and Mental Health. [online] Available at: www.ash.org.uk/category/information-and-resources/fact-sheets (accessed 19 June 2018).

Adler, L, Peselow, E, Rosenthal, M and Angrist, B (1993) A Controlled Comparison of the Effects of Propranolol, Benztropine, and Placebo on Akathisia. *Psychopharmacology Bulletin*, 29: 283–6.

AIHW: Australian Institute of Health and Welfare (2013) National Drug Strategy Household Survey. Canberra: AIHW. [online] Available at: www.aihw.gov.au/reports/illicit-use-of-drugs/national-drug-strategy-household-survey-detailed-report-2013/contents/table-of-contents (accessed 13 July 2018).

Allison, D B, Newcomer, J W, Dunn, A L, et al (2009) Obesity among Those with Mental Disorders: A National Institute of Mental Health Meeting Report. *American Journal of Preventative Medicine*, 36(4): 341–50.

Alvir, J M, Lieberman, J A, Safferman, A Z, Schwimmer, J L and Schaaf, J A (1993) Clozapine-Induced Agranulocytosis: Incidence and Risk Factors in the United States. *New England Journal of Medicine*, 329: 162–7.

Andrews, G and Jenkins, R (1999) *Management of Mental Disorders* (2nd ed). Sydney: World Health Organisation Collaborating Centre for Mental Health and Substance Abuse.

Anghelescu, I and Wolf, J (2004) Successful Switch to Aripiprazole After Induction of Hyperprolactinemia by Ziprasidone: A Case Report. *Journal of Clinical Psychiatry*, 65: 1286–7.

Atlantis, E and Baker, M (2008) Obesity Effects on Depression: Systematic Review of Epidemiological Studies. *International Journal of Obesity*, 32(6): 881–91.

Ballard, C, Hanney, M L, Theodoulou, M, et al (2009) The Dementia Antipsychotic Withdrawal Trial (DART-AD): Long-Term Follow-Up of a Randomised Placebo-Controlled Trial. *The Lancet Neurological*, 8: 151–7.

Ballon, J S, Pajvani U B, Mayer L E, et al (2018) Pathophysiology of Drug Induced Weight and Metabolic Effects: Findings from an RCT in Healthy Volunteers Treated with Olanzapine, Iloperidone, or Placebo. *Journal of Psychopharmacology*, 32(5): 533–40.

Barchas J D and Altemus, M (1999) Monoamine Hypotheses of Mood Disorders. In Siegel G J, Agranoff B W, Albers R W, et al (eds) *Basic Neurochemistry: Molecular, Cellular and Medical Aspects* (6th ed). Philadelphia: Lippincott-Raven. [online] Available at: www.ncbi.nlm.nih.gov/books/NBK28257 (accessed 11 July 2018).

Baskak B, Atbasoglu, E C, Ozguven, H D, Saka, M C and Gogus, A K (2007) The Effectiveness of Intramuscular Biperiden in Acute Akathisia: A Double-Blind, Randomized, Placebo-Controlled Study. *Journal of Clinical Psychopharmacology*, 27: 289–94.

Beasley, C M, Dellva, M, Tamura, R, et al (1999) Randomised Double-Blind Comparison of the Incidence of Tardive Dyskinesia in Patients With Schizophrenia During Long-Term Treatment with Olanzapine or Haloperidol. *British Journal of Psychiatry*, 174: 23–35.

Bhui, K, Weich, S and Lloyd, K (1998) *Pocket Psychiatry*. London: Mackays of Chatham.

Bjornsson, E (2008) Hepatotoxicity Associated with Antiepileptic Drugs. *Acta Neurology Scandinavica*, 118: 281–90.

Blow, W T (2011) *The Biological Basis of Mental Health Nursing* (2nd ed). London: Routledge.

Bond, A J (1998) Drug-Induced Behavioural Disinhibition Incidence, Mechanisms and Therapeutic Implications. *CNS Drugs*, 9: 41–57.

Bradley, E, Blackshaw, C and Nolan, P (2006) Nurse Lecturers' Observations on Aspects of Nurse Prescribing Training. *Nurse Education Today*, 26: 538–44.

Bray, G A (2004) Medical Consequences of Obesity. *Journal of Clinical Endocrinology*, 89: 2583–9.

Brent, B K, Thermenos, H W, Keshavan, M S and Seidman, L J (2013) Gray Matter Alterations in Schizophrenia High-Risk Youth and Early Onset Schizophrenia: A Review of Structural MRI Findings. *Child Adolescent Psychiatric Clinics of North America*, 22(4): 689–714.

British National Formulary (2014) *Publishing and RPS Publishing*. London: BNF.

British National Formulary and National Institute for Health and Care Excellence (BNF) (2018a) Antidepressant Drugs: Overview. [online] Available at: www.bnf.nice.org.uk/treatment-summary/antidepressant-drugs.html (accessed 3 March 2018).

British National Formulary and National Institute for Health and Clinical Excellence (BNF) (2018b) Clozapine. [online] Available at: www.bnf.nice.org.uk/drug/clozapine.html (accessed 19 June 2018).

British National Formulary and National Institute for Health and Clinical Excellence (BNF) (2018c) Lithium Carbonate. [online] Available at: www.bnf.nice.org.uk/drug/lithium-carbonate.html#monitoringRequirements (accessed 19 June 2018).

British National Formulary and National Institute for Health and Clinical Excellence (BNF) (2018d) Sodium valproate; MHRA/CHM advice: Valproate and Risk of Abnormal Pregnancy Outcomes. [online] Available at: www.bnf.nice.org.uk/drug/sodium-valproate.html (accessed 19 June 2018).

Brown, S, Kim, M, Mitchell, C and Inskip, H (2010) Twenty-Five-Year Mortality of a Community Cohort with Schizophrenia. *British Journal of Psychiatry*, 196: 116–21.

Buckley, N A and Sanders, A (2000) Cardiovascular Adverse Effects of Antipsychotic Drugs. *Drug Safety*, 23(3): 215–28.

Bullock, R, Touchon, J, Bergman, H, et al (2005) Rivastigmine and Donepezil Treatment in Moderate to Moderately Severe Alzheimer's Disease Over a 2-Year Period. *Current Medical Research and Opinion*, 21: 1317–27.

Cabrera, L S, Santana, A S, Robaina, P E and Palacios, M S (2010) Paradoxical Reaction to Midazolam Reversed with Flumazenil. *Journal of Emergencies, Trauma and Shock*, 3(3): 307.

Calabrese, J R and Delucchi, G A (1990) Spectrum of Efficacy of Valproate in 55 Patients with Rapid Cycling. *American Journal of Psychiatry*, 147(4): 431–4.

Campion, J, Hewitt, J, Shiers, D and Taylor, D (2017) *Pharmacy Guidance on Smoking and Mental Disorder – 2017 Update*. London: Royal College of Psychiatrists, National Pharmacy Association and Royal Pharmaceutical Society (RPS).

Care Quality Commission (2017) *Brief Guide: Physical Healthcare in Mental Health Settings*. London: Care Quality Commission.

Carnahan, R M, Lund, B C, Perry, P J and Chrischilles, E A (2004) The Concurrent Use of Anticholinergics and Cholinesterase Inhibitors: Rare Event or Common Practice? *Journal of American Geriatric Society*, 52: 2082–7.

Castelnovo, A, Ferrarelli, F and D'Agostino, A (2015) Schizophrenia: From Neurophysiological Abnormalities to Clinical Symptoms. *Frontiers in Psychology*, 6: 478.

Cavallaro, R, Cocchi, F, Angelone, S M, Lattuada, E and Smeraldi, E (2004) Cabergoline Treatment of Risperidone-Induced Hyperprolactinemia: A Pilot Study. *Journal of Clinical Psychiatry*, 65: 187–90.

Chen, J J, Ondo, W G, Dashtipour, K and Swope, D M (2012) Tetrabenazine for the Treatment of Hyperkinetic Movement Disorders: A Review of the Literature. *Clinical Therapeutics*, 34(7): 1487–504.

Chen, Y, Jiang, Y and Mao, Y (2009) Association Between Obesity and Depression in Canadians. *Journal of Women's Health*, 18(10): 1687–92.

Crump, C, Winkleby, M A and Sundquist, K (2013) Comorbidities and Mortality in Persons with Schizophrenia: A Swedish National Cohort Study. *American Journal of Psychiatry,* 170: 324–33.

Correll, C U, Parikh, U H, Mughal, T, et al (2005) Body Composition Changes Associated with Second Generation Antipsychotics. *Biological Psychiatry,* 7: 36.

Correll, C U, Lencz, T and Malhotra, A (2011) Antipsychotic Drugs and Obesity. *Trends in Molecular Medicine.* 17: 97–107.

Cowan, C and Oakley, C (2007) Leukopenia and Neutropenia Induced by Quetiapine. *Neuropsychopharmacology Biological Psychiatry,* 31: 292–4.

Cuellar, A K, Johnson, S L and Winters, R (2005) Distinctions Between Bipolar and Unipolar Depression. *Clinical Psychology Review,* 25(3): 307–39.

Culpepper, L (2010) The Role of Primary Care Clinicians in Diagnosing and Treating Bipolar Disorder. *Primary Care Companion to The Journal of Clinical Psychiatry,* 12(Suppl 1): 4–9.

Dalili, H, Nayeri, F, Shariat, M and Asgarzadeh, L (2015) Lamotrigine Effects on Breastfed Infants. *Acta Med Iran,* 53(7): 393–4.

De Abreu, L N, Lafer, B, Baca-Garcia, E and Oquendo, M A (2009) Suicidal Ideation and Suicide Attempts in Bipolar Disorder Type I: An Update for the Clinician. *Revista Brasileira de Psiquiatria,* 31(3): 271–80.

De Hert, M, Dekker, J M, Wood, D, et al (2009) Cardiovascular Disease and Diabetes in People with Severe Mental Illness Position Statement from the European Psychiatric Association (EPA), Supported by the European Association for the Study of Diabetes (EASD) and the European Society of Cardiology (ESC). *European Psychiatry,* 2(6): 412–24.

De Hert, M, Cohen, D, Bobes, J, et al (2011) Physical Illness in Patients With Severe Mental Disorders. II. Barriers to Care, Monitoring and Treatment Guidelines, Plus Recommendations at the System and Individual Level. *World Psychiatry,* 10: 138–51.

Department of Health (2017) *Towards a Smoke-Free Generation: Tobacco Control Plan For England.* London: DH. Stationery Office.

Di Venanzio, C, Marini, C, Santini, I, et al (2015) Severe Long Term Chronic Complications of Neuroleptic Malignant Syndrome: A Case Report. *Journal of Psychopathology,* 21: 97–100.

Dougherty, L, Lister, S and West-Oram, A (eds) (2015) *The Royal Marsden Manual of Clinical Nursing Procedures* (9th ed). Chichester: Wiley Blackwell.

Duggal, H S, Gates, C and Pathak, P C (2004) Olanzapine-Induced Neutropenia: Mechanism and Treatment. *Journal of Clinical Psychopharmacology,* 24: 234–5.

Dunstan, S (2010) *General Lifestyle Survey Overview: A Report on the 2010 General Lifestyle Survey.* Newport: Office for National Statistics.

Duncan, C, Yarwood, T and Bowden, R (2004) MIMS Handbook of Psychiatry. London: Haymarket Publishing Services Ltd.

Emre, M, Aarsland, D, Albanese, A, et al (2004) Rivastigmine for Dementia Associated with Parkinson's Disease. *New England Journal of Medicine,* 351: 2509–18.

Enger, C, Weatherby, L, Reynolds, R F, Glasser, D B and Walker, A W (2004) Serious Cardiovascular Events and Mortality Among Patients With Schizophrenia. *Journal of Nervous and Mental Disease,* 192(1): 19–27.

Fabricatore, A N and Wadden, T A (2006) Obesity. *Annual Review of Clinical Psychology,* 2: 357–77.

Farlow, M R and Cumming, J L (2007) Effective Pharmacologic Management of Alzheimer's Disease. *American Journal of Medicine,* 120: 388–97.

Farlow, M R and Shamliyan, T A (2017) Benefits and Harms of Atypical Antipsychotics for Agitation in Adults with Dementia. *European Neuropsychopharmacology,* 27(3): 217–31.

Fava, M (2000) New Approaches to the Treatment of Refractory Depression. *Journal of Clinical Psychiatry,* 61: 26–32.

Fisher, C and Boderick, W (2003) Sodium Valproate or Valproate Semi-Sodium: Is There a Difference in the Treatment of Bipolar Disorder? *Psychiatric Bulletin,* 27: 446–8.

Frankle, W G, Gil, R, Hackett, E, et al (2004) Occupancy of Dopamine D2 Receptors by the Atypical Antipsychotic Drugs Risperidone and Olanzapine: Theoretical Implications. *Psychopharmacology,* 175: 473–80.

Frodl, T (2017) Recent Advances in Predicting Responses to Antidepressant Treatment. *F1000Research,* 6: 619.

Gallinat, J, McMahon, K, Kühn, S, Schubert, F and Schaefer, M (2016) Cross-Sectional Study of Glutamate in the Anterior Cingulate and Hippocampus in Schizophrenia. *Schizophrenia Bulletin,* 42(2): 425–33.

Gauthier, S and Molinuevo, J L (2013) Benefits of Combined Cholinesterase Inhibitor and Memantine Treatment in Moderate-Severe Alzheimer's Disease. *Alzheimer's & Dementia,* 9(3): 326–31.

Geddes, J R, Burgess, S, Hawton, K, Jamison, K and Goodwin, G M (2004) Long-Term Lithium Therapy for Bipolar Disorder: Systematic Review and Meta-Analysis of Randomized Controlled Trials. *American Journal of Psychiatry,* 161: 217–22.

Gejman, P, Sanders, A and Duan, J (2010) The Role of Genetics in the Etiology of Schizophrenia. *The Psychiatric Clinics of North America,* 33(1): 35–66.

Goff, D C, Cather, C, Evins, A E, et al (2005) Medical Morbidity and Mortality in Schizophrenia: Guidelines for Psychiatrists. *Journal of Clinical Psychiatry,* 66(2):183–94.

Grabe, H J, Wolf, T, Gratz, C and Laux, G (1999) The Influence of Clozapine and Typical Neuroleptics on Information Processing of the Central Nervous System Under Clinical Conditions in Schizophrenic Disorders: Implications for Fitness to Drive. *Neuropsychobiology,* 40: 196–201.

Greil, W, Haag, H, Rossnagl, G and Ruther, F (1984) Effect of Anticholinergics on Tardive Dyskinesia: A Controlled Discontinuation Study. *British Journal of Psychiatry,* 145: 304–10.

Gundersen, C, Mahatmya, D, Garasky, S and Lohman, B (2010) Linking Psychosocial Stressors and Childhood Obesity. *Obesity Reviews,* 3(10).

Haas, M, Eerdekens, M, Kushner, S, et al (2009) Efficacy, Safety and Tolerability of Two Risperidone Dosing Regimens in Adolescent Schizophrenia: Double-Blind Study. *British Journal of Psychiatry,* 194: 158–64.

Haas, S J, Hill, J, Krum, H, et al (2007) Clozapine-Associated Myocarditis: A Review of 116 Cases of Suspected Myocarditis Associated with the Use of Clozapine in Australia during 1993–2003. *Drug Safety,* 30(1): 47–57.

Haddad, P M and Wieck, A (2004) Antipsychotic-Induced Hyperprolactinaemia: Mechanisms, Clinical Features and Management. *Drugs,* 64: 2291–314.

Hansen, T E, Casey, D E and Hoffman, W F (1997) Neuroleptic Intolerance. *Schizophrenia Bulletin,* 23: 567–83.

Harmer, C J, Goodwin, G M and Cowen, P J (2009) Why Do Antidepressants Take So Long to Work? A Cognitive Neuropsychological Model of Antidepressant Drug Action. *The British Journal of Psychiatry,* 195 (2): 102–8.

Hata, K, Iida, J, Iwasaka, H, Negoro, H and Kishimoto, T (2003) Association Between Minor Physical Anomalies and Lateral Ventricular Enlargement in Childhood and Adolescent Onset Schizophrenia. *Acta Psychiatrica Scandinavica,* 108(2): 147–51.

Heimpel, H (1996) When Should a Clinician Suspect a Drug-Induced Blood Dyscrasia, and How Should He Proceed? *European Journal of Haematology,* 57(60): 11–5.

Hernandez, R K, Farwell, W, Cantor, M D and Lawler, E V (2009) Cholinesterase Inhibitors and Incidence of Bradycardia in Patients with Dementia in the Veteran's Affairs New England Healthcare System. *Journal of American Geriatric Society*, 57: 1997–2003.

Herrmann, N, Gill, S S, Bell, C M, et al (2007) A Population-Based Study of Cholinesterase Inhibitor Use for Dementia. *Journal of American Geriatric Society*, 55: 1517–23.

Holland, L, Floyd, E and Soames, S (2018) *The Nurse's Guide to Mental Health Medicines*. London: SAGE Publishers.

Holmes, C, Wilkinson, D, Dean, C, et al (2004) The Efficacy of Donepezil in the Treatment of Neuropsychiatric Symptoms in Alzheimer Disease. *Neurology*, 27: 214–9.

Hu, W, MacDonald, M L, Elswick, D E and Sweet, R A (2015) The Glutamate Hypothesis of Schizophrenia: Evidence From Human Brain Tissue Studies. *Annals of the New York Academy of Sciences*, 1338(1): 38–57.

Iqbal, N, Lambert, T and Masand, P (2007) Akathisia: Problem of History or Concern of Today. *CNS Spectrums*, 12: 1–13.

Jacobs, G D, Pace-Schott, E F, Stickgold, R and Otto, M W (2004) Cognitive Behaviour Therapy and Pharmacotherapy for Insomnia: A Randomized Controlled Trial and Direct Comparison. *Archives of Internal Medicine*, 164: 1888–96.

Jamora, D, Lim, S, Pan, A, Tan, L and Tan, E (2007) Valproate Induced Parkinsonism in Epilepsy Patients. *Movement Disorder*, 22: 130–3.

Jankovic, J and Beach, J (1997) Long-Term Effects of Tetrabenazine in Hyperkinetic Movement Disorders. *Neurology*, 48: 358–62.

Javitt, D C (2007) Glutamate and Schizophrenia: Phencyclidine, N-methyl-D-aspartate Receptors, and Dopamine-Glutamate Interactions, in Integrating the Neurobiology of Schizophrenia. *International Review of Neurobiology*, 78: 59–108.

Jenkins, T A, Nguyen, J C D, Polglaze, K E, and Bertrand, P P (2016) Influence of Tryptophan and Serotonin on Mood and Cognition with a Possible Role of the Gut-Brain Axis. *Nutrients*, 8(1): 56.

Jick, H, Kaye, J A and Jick, S S (2004) Antidepressants and the Risk of Suicidal Behaviours. *Journal of American Medical Association*, 292: 338–43.

Joan, M D, Prasad, R P and Teri, L G (2006) Careful Monitoring for Agranulocytosis During Carbamazepine Treatment: Primary Care Companion. *Journal of Clinical Psychiatry*, 8(5): 310–31.

Johnston, A M and Eagles, J M (1999) Lithium-Associated Clinical Hypothyroidism. Prevalence and Risk Factors. *British Journal of Psychiatry*, 175: 336–9.

Joseph, J (2003) *The Gene Illusion: Genetic Research in Psychiatry and Psychology Under the Microscope*. Herefordshire: PCCS Books.

Juurlink, D N, Mamdani, M M, Kopp, A, et al (2004) Drug-Induced Lithium Toxicity in the Elderly: A Population-Based Study. *Journal of American Geriatric Society*, 52: 794–8.

Kane, J M, Fleischhacker, W W, Hansen, L, et al (2009) Akathisia: An Updated Review Focusing on Second Generation Antipsychotics. *Journal of Clinical Psychiatry*, 70: 627–43.

Katsiki, N, Apostolos, I H and Dimitri, P M (2011) Naltrexone Sustained-Release (SR) + Bupropion SR Combination Therapy for the Treatment of Obesity: 'A new kid on the block'? *Annals of Medicine*, 43(4): 249–58.

Khasawneh, F T and Shankar, G S (2013) Minimizing Cardiovascular Adverse Effects of Atypical Antipsychotic Drugs in Patients with Schizophrenia. *Cardiology Research and Practice*, 9(3): 326–31.

Kinon, B J, Gilmore, J A, Liu, H and Halbreich, U M (2003) Hyperprolactinemia in Response to Antipsychotic Drugs: Characterization Across Comparative Clinical Trials. *Psychoneuroendocrinology*, 28: 69–82.

Kirkbride, J B, Errazuriz, A, Croudace, T J, et al (2012) Incidence of Schizophrenia and Other Psychoses in England, 1950–2009: A Systematic Review and Meta-Analyses. *PloS One*, 7(3): e31660.

Kivimaki, M, Batty, G, Singh-Manoux, A, et al (2009) Association Between Common Mental Disorder and Obesity Over the Adult Life Course. *British Journal of Psychiatry*, 195(2): 149–55.

Knable, M B, Egan, M F, Heinz, A, et al (1997) Altered Dopaminergic Function and Negative Symptoms in Drug-Free Patients With Schizphrenia. [123I]-Iodobenzamide SPECT Study. *British Journal of Psychiatry*, 171: 574–7.

Koliscak, L and Makela, E (2009) Selective Serotonin Reuptake Inhibitor Induced Akathisia. *Journal of American Pharmacological Association*, 49: e28–36.

Krüger, S (2007) Dual Acting Antidepressants: What Are the Key Aspects in Terms of Short and Long-Term Clinical Efficacy? *BMC Psychiatry*, 7(Suppl 1): S71.

Lacro, J P, Dunn, L B, Dolder, C R, Leckband, S G and Jeste, D V (2002) Prevalence of and Risk Factors for Medication Nonadherence in Patients With Schizophrenia: A Comprehensive Review of Recent Literature. *Journal of Clinical Psychiatry*, 63: 892–909.

Lakhan, S E, Caro, M and Hadzimichalis, N (2013) NMDA Receptor Activity in Neuropsychiatric Disorders. *Frontiers in Psychiatry*, 4: 52.

Lam, D H, Hayward, P, Watkins, E R, Wright, K and Sham, P (2005) Relapse Prevention in Patients with Bipolar Disorder: Cognitive Therapy Outcome After 2 Years. *Amerian Journal of Psychiatry*, 162: 324.

Laoutidis, C G and Luckhaus, C (2014) 5-HT2A Receptor Antagonists for the Treatment of Neuroleptic-Induced Akathisia: A Systematic Review and Meta-Analysis. *International Journal of Neuropsychopharmac ology*, 17(5): 823–40.

Lester, H, Shiers, D and Rafi, I (2012) *Positive Cardiometabolic Health Resource: An Intervention Framework for Patients with Psychosis on Antipsychotic Medication*. Royal College of Psychiatrists: London.

Lima, A R, Soares-Weiser, K, Bacaltchuk, J and Barnes, T (2002) Benzodiazepines for Neuroleptic-Induced Acute Akathisia. *The Cochrane Database of Systematic Reviews*, (1): CD001950.

Lopez, O L, Becker, J T, Wahed, A S, et al (2009) Long-Term Effects of the Concomitant Use of Memantine with Cholinesterase Inhibition in Alzheimer Disease. *Journal of Neurology Neurosurgical Psychiatry*, 80: 600–7.

López-Pousa, S, Garre-Olmo, J and Vilalta-Franch, J (2007) Galantamine Versus Donepezil in the Treatment of Alzheimer's Disease. *Reviews of Neurology*, 44: 677–84.

Louza, M R and Bassitt, D P (2005) Maintenance Treatment of Severe Tardive Dyskinesia with Clozapine: Five Years Follow-Up. *Journal of Clinical Psychopharmacology*, 25: 180–2.

Luppino, F S, de Wit, L M, Bouvy, P F, et al (2010) Overweight, Obesity, and Depression: A Systematic Review and Meta-Analysis of Longitudinal Studies. *Archives of General Psychiatry*, 67(3): 220–9.

Ma, J and Xiao, L (2010) Obesity and Depression in US Women: Results from the 2005–2006 National Health and Nutritional Examination Survey. *Obesity*, 18(2): 347–53.

Mailman, R B and Murthy, V (2010) Third Generation Antipsychotic Drugs: Partial Agonism or Receptor Functional Selectivity? *Current Pharmaceutical Design*, 16: 488–501.

Malhi, G S, Adams, D and Berk, M (2009) Is Lithium in a Class of its Own? A Brief Profile of its Clinical Use. *Australia New Zealand Journal of Psychiatry*, 43: 1093–104.

Malhi, G S, Adams, D and Berk, M (2010) The Pharmacological Treatment of Bipolar Disorder in Primary Care. *Medical Journal of Australia*, 193: S24–30.

Malhi, G S, Tanious, M, Das, P, Coulston, C M and Berk, M (2013) Potential Mechanisms of Action of Lithium in Bipolar Disorder: Current Understanding. *CNS Drugs*, 27(2): 135–53.

Mancuso, C E, Tanzi, M G and Gabay, M (2004) Paradoxical Reactions to Benzodiazepines: Literature Review and Treatment Options. *Pharmacotherapy,* 24(9): 1177–85.

Markowitz, S, Friedman, M A and Arent, S M (2008) Understanding the Relation Between Obesity and Depression: Causal Mechanisms and Implications for Treatment. *Clinical Psychology: Science and Practice*, 15(1): 1–20.

McGrath, J and Soares-Weiser, K (2011) Vitamin E for Neuroleptic-Induced Tardive Dyskinesia. *The Cochrane Database of Systematic Reviews*, 16(2): CD000209.

McKeith, I, Del Ser, T, Spano, P, et al (2000) Efficacy of Rivastigmine in Dementia with Lewy Bodies: A Randomised, Double-Blind, Placebo-Controlled International Study. *Lancet*, 356: 2031–6.

McShane, R, Areosa, S A and Minakaran, N (2006) Memantine for Dementia. *The Cochrane Database of Systematic Reviews*, 19(2): CD003154.

Medicines and Healthcare Products Regulatory Agency (MHRA) (2008) *Medicine and Medical Devices Regulation*. London: MHRA.

Medicines and Healthcare Products Regulation Agency (MHRA) (2014) *Valproate: Patient Guide*. London: MHRA.

Medicines Healthcare Products Regulatory Agency (MHRA) (2018) *Drug Safety Update: Valproate Medicines* (Epilim▼, Depakote▼). [online] Available at: www.gov.uk/drug-safety-update/valproate-medicines-epilim-depakote-contraindicated-in-women-and-girls-of-childbearing-potential-unless-conditions-of-pregnancy-prevention-programme-are-met (accessed 24 April 2018).

Mental Health Foundation (2016) *Fundamental Facts About Mental Health*. London: Mental Health Foundation.

Mental Health Taskforce to the NHS England (2016) *The Five Year Forward View for Mental Health*. [online] Available at: www.england.nhs.uk/wp-content/uploads/2016/02/Mental-Health-Taskforce-FYFV-final.pdf (accessed 12 June 2018).

Merikangas, K R, Jin, R, He, J, et al (2011) Prevalence and Correlates of Bipolar Spectrum Disorder in the World Mental Health Survey Initiative. *Archives of General Psychiatry*, 68(3): 241–51.

Mert, D G, Turgut, N H, Kelleci, M and Semiz, M (2015) Perspectives on Reasons of Medication Nonadherence in Psychiatric Patients. *Patient Preference and Adherence*, 9: 87–93.

Messias, E L, Chen, C Y and Eaton, W W (2007) Epidemiology of Schizophrenia: Review of Findings and Myths. *North American Clinical Psychiatry*, 30: 323.

Meyer, J H, McNeely, H E, Sagrati, S, et al (2006) Elevated Putamen D2 Receptor Binding Potential in Major Depression with Motor Retardation: An [11C] Raclopride Positron Emission Study. *American Journal of Psychiatry*, 163(9): 1594–1602.

Mimidis, K, Papadopoulos, V and Thomopoulos, K (2003) Prolongation of the QTc Interval in Patients with Cirrhosis. *Annals of Gastroenterology*, 16(2): 155–8.

Mind (2014) Antidepressants A–Z: Provides Detailed Information on all Antidepressant Drugs Currently Available in the UK. [online] Available at: www.mind.org.uk/information-support/drugs-and-treatments/antidepressants-a-z/#.WyBndoVOLVI (accessed 12 June 2018).

Moghaddam, B and Javitt, D (2012) From Revolution to Evolution: The Glutamate Hypothesis of Schizophrenia and Its Implication for Treatment. *Neuropsychopharmacology*, 37(1): 4–15.

Mond, J M and Baune, B T (2009) Overweight, Medical Comorbidity and Health-Related Quality of Life in a Community Sample of Women and Men. *Obesity*, 17(8): 1627–34.

Morrato, E, Newcomer, J W, Kamat, S, Baser, O and Cuffel, B (2009) Metabolic Screening After the American Diabetes Association's Consensus Statement on Antipsychotic Drugs and Diabetes. *Diabetes Care*, 32: 1037–42.

Morrato, E H, Druss, B, Hartung, D M, et al (2010) Metabolic Testing Rates in 3 State Medicaid Programs After FDA Warnings and ADA/APA Recommendations for Second Generation Antipsychotic Drugs. *Archives of General Psychiatry*, 67: 17–24.

Mutsatsa, S (2015) *Physical Healthcare and Promotion in Mental Health Nursing*. London: SAGE Publishers.

Mwebe, H (2017) Physical Health Monitoring in Mental Health Settings: A Study Exploring Mental Health Nurses' Views of Their Role. *Journal of Clinical Nursing*, 19–20: 3067–78.

Mwebe, H (2018) Serious Mental Illness and Smoking Cessation, *British Journal of Mental Health Nursing*, 7(1): 39–46.

Nadkarni, P, Jayaram, M, Nadkarni, S, Rattehalli, R and Adams, C E (2015) Rapid Tranquillisation: A Global Perspective. *British Journal of Psychiatry International*, 12(4): 100–2.

Nash, M (2011) *Physical Health and Well-Being in Mental Health Nursing: Clinical Skills for Practice*. London: Open University Press.

National Institute for Health and Care Excellence (NICE) (2011) Generalised Anxiety Disorder and Panic Disorder in Adults: Management. Clinical Guidance 113. [online] Available at: www.nice.org.uk/guidance/cg113 (accessed 12 June 2018).

National Institute for Health and Clinical Excellence (2015) Violence and Aggression the Short-Term Management in Mental Health, Health and Community Settings, NICE Guideline 10. [online] Available at: www.nice.org.uk/guidance/ng10 (accessed 14 March 2018).

National Institute for Health and Care Excellence (NICE) (2018a) Bipolar Disorder: Assessment and Management, Clinical Guidance 185. [online] Available at: www.nice.org.uk/guidance/cg185 (accessed 12 June 2018).

National Institute for Health and Care Excellence (NICE) (2018b) Depression in Adults: Recognition and Management, Clinical Guidance 90. [online] Available at: www.nice.org.uk/guidance/cg90 (accessed 12 June 2018).

National Institute for Health and Clinical Excellence (2018c) Dementia: Assessment, Management and Support for People Living with Dementia and Their Carers, National Guidance 97. [online] Available at: www.nice.org.uk/guidance/ng97/chapter/Recommendations#pharmacological-interventions-for-dementia (accessed 13 July 2018).

National Institute of Mental Health (2016) Brain Basics. NIMH. [online] Available at: www.nimh.nih.gov/health/educational-resources (accessed 15 June 2018).

National Obesity Observatory (2011) *Obesity and Mental Health*. London: Public Health England.

Nemeroff, C B, Schatsberg, A F, Goldstein, D J, et al (2002) Duloxetine for the Treatment of Major Depressive Disorder. *Psychopharmacology Bulletin*, 36(4): 106–32.

Newcomer, J W (2005) Second Generation (Atypical Antipsychotics) and Metabolic Effects: A Comprehensive Literature Review. *CNS Drugs*, 19(Suppl 1): 1–93.

NHS England (2014) Commissioning for Quality and Innovation (CQUIN): 2014/15 Guidance. [online] Available at: www.england.nhs.uk/wp-content/uploads/2014/02/sccquin-guid.pdf (accessed 8 July 2018).

Nierenberg, A A and DeCocco, L M (2001) Definitions of Antidepressant Treatment Response, Remission, Nonresponse, Partial Response, and Other Relevant Outcomes: A Focus on Treatment-Resistant Depression. *Journal of Clinical Psychiatry*, 62(Suppl 16): 5–9.

Nooijen, P M, Carvalho, F and Flanagan, R J (2011) Haematological Toxicity of Clozapine and Some Other Drugs Used in Psychiatry. *Human Psychopharmacology*, 26: 112–19.

Nose, M, Barbui, C and Tansella, M (2003) How Often Do Patients with Psychosis Fail to Adhere to Treatment Programmes? A Systematic Review. *Psychological Medicine*, 33: 1149–60.

Nursing and Midwifery Council (NMC) (2008) Standards for Medicines Management. [online] Available at: www.nmc.org.uk/globalassets/sitedocuments/standards/nmc-standards-for-medicines-management.pdf (accessed 19 June 2018).

Nursing and Midwifery Council (NMC) (2015) *The Code: Standards of Conduct, Performance and Ethics for Nurses and Midwives*. London: NMC.

Nursing and Midwifery Council (NMC) (2015b) *The Code: Standards for Medicine Management.* London: NMC.

Nursing and Midwifery Council (NMC) (2017) *Educational Framework. Standards for Education and Training: Draft for Consultation.* London: NMC.

Nursing and Midwifery Council (NMC) (2018) Standards For Medicines Management. [online] Available at: www.nmc.org.uk/standards/standards-for-post-registration/standards-for-medicines-management (accessed 19 June 2018).

Office for National Statistics (ONS) (2016) General Household Survey. Statistical Bulletin. [online] Available at: www.ons.gov.uk (accessed 15 June 2018).

Offredy, M, Kendall, S and Goodman, C (2008) The Use of Cognitive Continuum Theory and Patient Scenarios to Explore Nurse Prescribers' Pharmacological Knowledge and Decision Making. *International Journal of Nursing Studies*, 45(6): 855–68.

Ondo, W, Hanna, P and Jankovic, J (1999) Tetrabenazine Treatment for Tardive Dyskinesia: Assessment by Randomized Videotape Protocol. *American Journal of Psychiatry*, 156: 1279–81.

Pacchiarotti, I, Baldessarini, R J, Nolen, W, et al (2013) The International Society for Bipolar Disorders (ISBD) Task-Force Report on Antidepressants Use in Bipolar Disorders. *American Journal of Psychiatry*, 170(11): 1249–62.

Pappagallo, M and Silva, R (2004) The Effect of Atypical Antipsychotic Agents on Prolactin Levels in Children and Adolescents. *Journal of Child and Adolescent Psychopharmacology*, 14(3): 359–71.

Peskind, E R, Potkin, S G and Pomara, N, et al (2006) Memantine Treatment in Mild to Moderate Alzheimer's Disease: A 24-Week Randomized, Controlled Trial. *American Journal of Geriatric Psychiatry*, 14: 704–15.

Phelan, M, Stradins, L and Morrison, S (2001) Physical Health of People With Severe Mental Illness. *British Medical Journal,* 322: 443–4.

Pies, R W (2005) *Handbook of Essential Psychopharmacology* (2nd ed). Washington, DC: American Psychiatric Press Inc.

Pilowsky, L S, Costa, D C, Ell, P J, et al (1993) Antipsychotic Medication, D2 Dopamine Receptor Blockade and Clinical Response: A 1231 IBZM SPET (Single Photon Emission Tomography) study. *Psychological Medicine*, 23: 791–9.

Poyurovsky, M, Pashinian, A, Weizman, R, Fuchs, C and Weizman, A (2006) Low-Dose Mirtazapine: A New Option in the Treatment of Antipsychotic-Induced Akathisia. A Randomized, Double-Blind, Placebo- and Propranolol-Controlled Trial. *Biological Psychiatry*, 59: 1071–7.

Poyurovsky, M and Weizman, A (2001) Serotonin-Based Pharmacotherapy for Acute Neuroleptic-Induced Akathisia: A New Approach to an Old Problem. *British Journal of Psychiatry*, 179: 4–8.

Poyurovsky, M (2010) Acute Antipsychotic-Induced Akathisia Revisited. *British Journal of Psychiatry*, 196(2): 89–91.

Quiroz, J A, Machado-Vieira, R, Zarate, J C A, et al (2010) Novel Insights into Lithium's Mechanism of Action: Neurotrophic and Neuroprotective Effects. *Neuropsychobiology*, 62(1): 50–60.

Rajappa, G C, Vig, S, Bevanaguddaiah, Y and Anadaswamy, T (2016) Efficacy of Pregabalin as Premedication for Post-Operative Analgesia in Vaginal Hysterectomy. *Anaesthesiology and Pain Medicine*, 6(3): e34591.

Rammes, G, Rupprecht, R, Ferrari, U, Zieglgansberger, W and Parsons, C G (2001) The N-Methyl-D-Aspartate Receptor Channel Blockers Memantine, MRZ 2/579 and Other Amino-Alkyl-Cyclohexanes Antagonise 5-HT (3) Receptor Currents in Cultured HEK-293 and N1E-115 Cell Systems in a Non-Competitive Manner. *Neuroscience Letters*, 306: 81–4.

Rana, A Q, Chaudry, Z M and Blanchet, P J (2013) New and Emerging Treatments for Symptomatic Tardive Dyskinesia. *Drug Design, Development and Therapy*, 6(7): 1329–40.

Rapp, P R and Bachevalier, J (2003) *Cognitive Development and Aging.* In Squire, L R, Bloom, F E, McConnell, S K, et al (eds) *Fundamental Neuroscience* (1167–99). New York: Academic Press.

Rickels, K and Schweizer, E (1998) Panic Disorder: Long-Term Pharmacotherapy and Discontinuation. *Journal of Clinical Psychopharmacology,* 18: 12–8.

Robinson, D S (2002) Monoamine Oxidase Inhibitors: A New Generation. *Psychopharmacology Bulletin,* 36(3): 124–38.

Robson, D and Gray, R (2007) Serious Mental Illness and Physical Health Problems: A Discussion Paper. *International Journal of Nursing Studies,* 44: 457–66.

Royal College of Psychiatrists (2012) *Report of the National Audit of Schizophrenia (NAS).* London: Healthcare Quality Improvement Partnership.

Royal College of Psychiatrists (2018) Depot Medication (Under Review). [online] Available at: www.rcpsych. ac.uk/healthadvice/treatmentsandwellbeing/depotmedication.aspx (accessed 10 April 2018).

Royal College of Physicians (2018) National Early Warning Score (NEWS 2): How NEWS Works. [online] Available at: www.rcplondon.ac.uk/projects/outputs/national-early-warning-score-news-2 (accessed 10 July 2018).

Royal Pharmaceutical Society (2016) *Prescribing Framework: A Competency Framework for all Prescribers.* London: RPS.

Rudolph, U, and Möhler, H (2014) GABAA Receptor Subtypes: Therapeutic Potential in Down Syndrome, Affective Disorders, Schizophrenia, and Autism. *Annual Review of Pharmacology and Toxicology,* 54: 483–507.

Satterwaite, T, Wolf, D, Rosenheck, R, Gur, R and Caroff, S (2008) A Meta-Analysis of the Risk of Acute Extrapyramidal Symptoms with Intramuscular Antipsychotics for the Treatment of Agitation. *Journal of Clinical Psychiatry,* 69: 1869–79.

Schatz, I J, Bannister, R, Freeman, R L, et al (1996) Consensus Statement on the Definition of Orthostatic Hypotension, Pure Autonomic Failure, and Multiple System Atrophy. *Journal of the Neurological Sciences,* 144(1–2): 218–19.

Scott, D and Happell, B (2011) The High Prevalence of Poor Physical Health and Unhealthy Lifestyle Behaviours in Individuals with Severe Mental Illness. *Issues in Mental Health Nursing,* 32: 589–97.

Scott, W N and McGrath, D (2009) *Nursing Pharmacology Made Incredibly Easy.* London: Lippincott Williams & Wilkins.

Seeman, P (2014) Clozapine, a Fast-Off-D2 Antipsychotic. *ACS Chemical Neuroscience,* 5(1): 24–9.

Severus, E and Bauer, M (2013) Diagnosing Bipolar Disorders in DSM-5. *International Journal of Bipolar Disorders,* 1: 14.

Silver, H, Geraisy, N and Schwartz, M (1995) No Difference in the Effect of Biperiden and Amantadine on Parkinsonian and Tardive Dyskinesia Type Involuntary Movements: A Double-Blind Crossover, Placebo-Controlled Study in Medicated Chronic Schizophrenic Patients. *Journal of Clinical Psychiatry,* 56: 167–70.

Simon, G E, Von Korff, M, Saunders, K, et al (2006) Association Between Obesity and Psychiatric Disorders in the US Adult Population. *Archives of General Psychiatry,* 63(7): 824–830.

Simpson, N, Maffei, A, Freeby, M, et al (2012) Dopamine-Mediated Autocrine Inhibitory Circuit Regulating Human Insulin Secretion In Vitro. *Molecular Endocrinology,* 26: 1757–72.

Sluys, M, Güzelcan, Y, Casteelen, G and de Haan, L (2004) Risperidone-Induced Leucopoenia and Neutropenia: A Case Report. *European Psychiatry,* 19(2): 117.

Smith, D, Dempster, C, Glanville, J, Freemantle, N and Anderson, I (2002) Efficacy and Tolerability of Venlafaxine Compared with Selective Serotonin Reuptake Inhibitors and Other Antidepressants: A Meta-Analysis. *British Journal of Psychiatry,* 180: 396–404.

Smith, S (2003) Effects of Antipsychotics on Sexual and Endocrine Function in Women: Implications for Clinical Practice. *Journal of Clinical Psychopharmacology*, 23: S27–S32.

Soreca, I, Frank, E and Kupfer, D J (2009) The Phenomenology of Bipolar Disorder: What Drives the High Rate of Medical Burden and Determines Long-Term Prognosis? *Depression and Anxiety*, 26(1): 73–82.

Spivak, B, Mester, R, Abesgaus, J, Wittenberg, N and Adlersberg, S (1997) Clozapine Treatment for Neuroleptic-Induced Tardive Dyskinesia, Parkinsonism, and Chronic Akathisia in Schizophrenic Patients. *Journal of Clinical Psychiatry*, 58: 318–22.

Stahl, S M (2006) *Essential Psychopharmacology: The Prescriber's Guide*. New York: Cambridge University Press.

Stahl, S M (2008) *Stahl's Essential Psychopharmacology: Neuroscientific Basis and Practical Applications*. New York: Cambridge University Press.

Stahl, S M (2013) *Stahl's Essential Psychopharmacology: Neuroscientific Basis and Practical Applications* (4th ed). New York: Cambridge University Press.

Stephen, L J (2003) Drug Treatment of Epilepsy in Elderly People: Focus on Valproic Acid. *Drugs Aging*, 20: 141–52.

Stockley's Drug Interactions (2018) Stockley's Interactions Checker. [online] Available at: https://about.medicinescomplete.com/publication/stockleys-interactions-checker (accessed 12 June 2018).

Südhof, T C (2004) The Synaptic Vesicle Cycles. *Annual Review of Neuroscience*, 27: 509–47.

Südhof, T C and Rothman, J E (2009) Membrane Fusion: Grappling With SNARE and SM Proteins. *Science*, 323: 474–7.

Sullivan, L E (2009) *The SAGE Glossary of the Social and Behavioural Sciences*. London: SAGE Publications.

Susce, M T, Villanueva, N, Diaz, F J and Deleon, J (2005) Obesity and Associated Complications in Patients with Severe Mental Illnesses: A Cross-Sectional Survey. *Clinical Psychiatry,* 66: 167–73.

Szatkowsk, L and McNeill, A (2015) Diverging Trends in Smoking Behaviours According to Mental Health Status. *Nicotine & Tobacco Research*, 3: 356–60.

Taylor, D and Duncan, D (1997) Doses of Carbamazepine and Valproate in Bipolar Affective Disorder. *Psychiatric Bulletin*, 21: 221–3.

Taylor, M J, Freemantle, N and Geddes, J R, et al (2006) Early Onset of Selective Serotonin Reuptake Inhibitor Antidepressant Action: Systematic Review and Meta-Analysis. *Archives of General Psychiatry*, 63: 1217–23.

Taylor, D, Paton, C and Kapur, S (2012) *The South London and Maudsley and Oxleas NHS Foundation Trusts Prescribing Guidelines* (10th ed). London: Wiley-Blackwell.

Taylor, D, Paton, C and Kerwin, R (2015) *The South London and Maudsley & Oxleas NHS Foundation Trusts Prescribing Guidelines* (12th ed). London: Wiley-Blackwell.

Tenback, D, van Harten, P, Slooff, C and Van, O J (2010) Incidence and Persistence of Tardive Dyskinesia and Extrapyramidal Symptoms in Schizophrenia. *Journal of Psychopharmacology*, 24: 1031–5.

Thase, M E, Trivedi, M H and Rush, A J (1995) MAOIs in the Contemporary Treatment of Depression. *Neuropsychopharmacology*, 12(3): 185–219.

Thase, M E (2003) Effectiveness of Antidepressants: Comparative Remission Rates. *Journal of Clinical Psychiatry*, 64(Suppl 2): 3–7.

The Health and Social Care Information Centre (2013) *Statistics on Obesity, Physical Activity and Diet: England*. London: The Health and Social Care Information Centre.

Tonda, M and Guthrie, S (1994) Treatment of Acute Neuroleptic-Induced Movement Disorders. *Pharmacotherapy*, 14: 543–60.

Tosh, G, Clifton, A V, Xia, J and White, M M (2014) General Physical Health Advice for People with Serious Mental Illness. *The Cochrane Database of Systematic Reviews*, (3): CD008567.

Trivedi, M H, Fava, M, Wisniewski, S R, et al (2006) Medication Augmentation After the Failure of SSRIs for Depression. *New England Journal of Medicine*, 354: 1243–52.

Tse, L, Barr, A M, Scarapicchia, V and Vila-Rodriguez, F (2015) Neuroleptic Malignant Syndrome: A Review from a Clinically Oriented Perspective. *Current Neuropharmacology*, 13(3): 395–406.

Van Rossum, J M (1966) The Significance of Dopamine-Receptor Blockade for the Action of Neuroleptic Drugs. In *Excerpta Medica International Congress Series No. 129 Proceedings of the Vth International Congress of the Collegium Internationale Neuropsychopharmacology Washington, 28–31*, 321–9.

Voulgari, C, Giannas, R, Paterakis, G, et al (2015) Clozapine-Induced Late Agranulocytosis and Severe Neutropenia Complicated with Streptococcus pneumonia, Venous Thromboembolism, and Allergic Vasculitis in Treatment-Resistant Female Psychosis. *Case Reports in Medicine*, 703218. [online] Available at: www.hindawi.com/journals/crim/2015/703218/cta (accessed 12 April 2018).

Waddell, L and Taylor, M (2008) GASS-Glasgow Antipsychotic Side-effect Scale. *Journal of Psychopharmacology*, 22(3): 238–43.

Wahl, R and Ostroff, R (2005) Reversal of Symptomatic Hyperprolactinemia by Aripiprazole. *American Journal of Psychiatry*, 162: 1542–3.

Wargo KA, Gupta R. Neuroleptic malignant syndrome: no longer exclusively a "neuroleptics" phenomenon. *Journal of Pharmaceutical Technology*, 21: 262–70.

Whishaw, I Q, Kolb, B and Teskey, C G (2016) *An Introduction to Brain and Behaviour* (5th ed). New York: Worth Publishers.

Winblad, B and Poritis, N (1999) Memantine in Severe Dementia: Results of the 9M-Best Study (Benefit and Efficacy in Severely Demented Patients During Treatment With Memantine). *International Journal of Geriatric Psychiatry*, 14: 135–46.

Wise, J (2017) Research News: Study Finds Lamotrigine to be Safe During Pregnancy. *British Medical Journal*. 359: j4827.

Woerner, M G, Alvir, J M, Saltz, B L, Lieberman, J A and Kane, J M (1998) Prospective Study of Tardive Dyskinesia in the Elderly: Rates and Risk Factors. *American Journal of Psychiatry*, 155(11): 1521–8.

World Health Organisation (2013) Premature Death Among People with Severe Mental Disorders: Information Sheet. [online] Available at: www.who.int/mental_health/management/info_sheet.pdf (accessed 15 June 2018).

World Health Organisation (2018) Premature Death Among People with Severe Mental Disorders: Information Sheet. [online] Available at: www.who.int/mental_health/management/info_sheet.pdf (accessed 8 July 2018).

Yassa, R and Bloom, D (1990) Lorazepam and Anticholinergics in Tardive Akathisia. *Biological Psychiatry*, 27: 463–4.

Youdim, M B, Edmondson, D and Tipton, K F (2006) The Therapeutic Potential of Monoamine Oxidase Inhibitors. *Nature Reviews of Neuroscience*, 7: 295–309.

Zhang, Z J, Tan, Q R, Tong, Y, et al (2008) The Effectiveness of Carbamazepine in Unipolar Depression: A Double-Blind, Randomized, Placebo-Controlled Study. *Journal of Affective Disorders*, 109: 91–7.

Zubin, J and Spring, B (1977) Vulnerability: A New View of Schizophrenia. *Journal of Abnormal Psychology*, 86(2): 103–24.

Index

You might also like:

Studying for your Nursing Degree by Jane Bottomley and Steven Pryjmachuk
ISBN 978-1-911106-91-3

Academic Writing and Referencing for your Nursing Degree by Jane Bottomley and
Steven Pryjmachuk ISBN 978-1-911106-95-1

Critical Thinking Skills for your Nursing Degree by Jane Bottomley and Steven
Pryjmachuk ISBN 978-1-912096-69-5

Communication Skills for your Nursing Degree by Jane Bottomley and Steven
Pryjmachuk ISBN 978-1-912096-65-7

Most of our titles are also available in a range of electronic formats. To order please go
to our website www.criticalpublishing.com or contact our distributor, NBN International,
10 Thornbury Road, Plymouth PL6 7PP, telephone 01752 202301 or email
orders@nbninternational.com.